The Complete Guide to Natural Toothache Remedies and Re-mineralization

Scott Rauvers

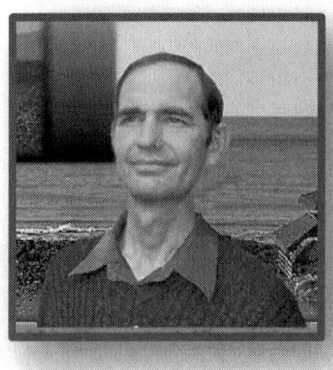

This book is dedicated to those that did not have the knowledge to avoid unnecessary root canals, so they may avoid unnecessary pain and expense in the future

Published by the Institute for Solar Studies

Read the first 3 chapters free at:
http://www.ez3dbiz.com/natural_cavity_remedies.

Copyright © November 2015 Scott Rauvers

All rights reserved.

The Complete Guide to Natural Toothache
Remedies and Re-mineralization

ISBN-13:
978-1512216882

ISBN-10:
1512216887

First Printing May 2015

Second Printing November 2015

Website: www.ez3dbiz.com

This book is available in Paperback, Nook and Kindle Versions.

Just enter the title into any Internet search box to locate these versions

A SPECIAL THANK YOU

Thank you the reader for being a part of those positively transforming the world of dentistry. This book is dedicated to those seeking how to tap into the power of nutritional wisdom to create healthy teeth and gums.

The sole purpose of this book is to empower those seeing alternatives to the dentist's drill and to help create a feeling of self confidence and comfort, knowing you hold the power to prevent cavities, re-mineralize your teeth and create lasting strong and healthy gums.

Use the wisdom in this book to: Avoid Unnecessary Root Canals, Learn to re-grow New Layers of Dentin on Exposed Enamel, Reverse Gum Disease, Heal Tooth Abscesses, Re-store your Hormones to Healthy Levels and visit a dentist only when absolutely necessary, This book can save you thousands of dollars and avoid wasted time on unnecessary dental procedures.

About the Author

Scott is the author of 4 books on longevity nutrition and anti aging focusing on Ayurvedic, European and Traditional Chinese Herbal Remedies.
(www.ez3dbiz.com/library.html)

Scott is also the founder of The Institute For Solar Studies On Behavior And Human Health, which studies non invasive methods of healing, giving people alternatives to painful and sometimes unnecessary surgery. Scott's latest book released in Spring of 2015 appropriately titled: The Complete Guide to Natural Toothache Remedies and Re-mineralization gives readers painless alternatives to root camels, herbal methods to relieve toothache and herbal remedies and mouth washes for sore, receding or infected gums. In his latest book Scott includes his own experiences of how these non-invasive methods have helped him and the many readers of his website avoid visiting the dentist altogether. This book is a golden gem if you live or spend time in locations you don't have access to a dentist or want to visit them unless absolutely necessary.

This book is part of our ongoing series about longevity using Nutraceuticals. Other books published by ez3dbiz.com include:

Released November 2013. – Foods, Herbs and Pharmaceuticals that Extend Lifespan. A Summary Of Over 200 Research Studies Proven To Lengthen Lifespan. ----This book has a special section on using Nutraceutical combinations to create stem cell longevity formulas that extend lifespan.

Released August 2014. – Anti Aging Nutrition Secrets. The Fountain of Youth Seekers Guide to Longevity–

Released August 2014. – A Centurion's Toolbox for Longevity Living Beyond 120 – 2nd Edition

Released September 2014. – Living Healthy Beyond 120, A Centurion's Plan for Longevity

Released July 2014. – The Emerald Tablets: The Keys of Life and Death by Thoth the Atlantean

CHAPTERS

Introduction — *ii*

How Mercury Damages the Body — *iii*

What is Dental Amalgam? — *iii*

Developed Countries that have Banned the Use of Mercury Fillings — *iv*

Why You Can Enjoy Better Health Using the Holistic Approach — *v*

Why Your Dentist Won't Share These Secrets With You — *vii*

A Special Message To Dentists — *ix*

When You, the Reader Should See A Dentist — *x*

Chapter 1 — *Page 13*

My Personal Story – — *Page 13*

Natural Tooth Repair Studies Performed By Dr. Weston Price – — *16*

Why Vegetarians
Get More Cavities — *18*

What is Vitamin K2? — *19*

Chapter 2 — *Page 23*

Simple and Effective Herbal Formulas for Teeth and Gums — *23*

Rosemary Gladstar's Healing Mouthwash — *23*

The Jean Valnet Remedy — *25*

A Preventive Health Mouth Wash — *26*

Jerthro Kloss Gum Healer and Mouth Rinse — *27*

An Ancient Chinese Herbal Remedy for Toothache — *28*

Michael Moore's Tooth Powder — *28*

Jared's Tooth Powder — *30*

Jakob Lorber's Tooth Remedy Powder — *31*

Ayurvedic Methods for Healing Toothache — *34*

Time Tested Chinese Herbal Remedies for Toothache — *35*

The Complete Guide to Natural Toothache Remedies and Re-mineralization

The Rehmannia Six Combination (Liu wei di huang wan)   *35*

The Niu Huang Jie Du Pian Formula   *37*

The Chinese herb Baizhi   *40*

The Chinese herb Xuchangqing   *40*

Native American Toothache Remedies   *41*

Using Watermelon Rind for Toothache Relief   *44*

How to Make Herbs into Fine Powder   *45*

Essential Oils and Herbs for Relief of Toothache   *46*

How to use Eucalyptus Oil   *50*

Natural Tea Contains High Amounts of Fluoride   *51*

Chapter 3   *Page 53*

Keeping the Gums Healthy   *Page 53*

Black or Green Tea for Healthy Gums   *54*

Herbal Remedies for Healthy Gums	57
Natural Methods That Tighten Gums	58
Chapter 4	Page 60
Herbs to Build Strong Teeth	60
Natural Non-Invasive Methods that Strengthen Teeth	62
The Best Tree Bark for Strong Teeth	65
Using Parsley For Re-Strengthening Loose Teeth	65
The Best Teas for Healthy Teeth and Gums	66
Methods to Tighten Gums	66
Natural Herbs for Oral Hygiene and Healthy Teeth	67
Using Coconut Oil to Dissolve Plaque	67
Chapter 5	Page 69
How Diet and Sugar Relate to Dental Health	69

The Complete Guide to Natural Toothache Remedies and Re-mineralization

A Simple Sugar Detox Plan	*69*
My Experience of Abstaining From Sugar	*70*
Dealing with Addictions to Sugar	*73*
Why You Crave Sugar	*73*
Methods that Help Eliminate Sugar Cravings	*74*
Chapter 6	*Page 76*
The Importance of Vitamins A, D and K	*76*
The Miracle of Vitamin K	*77*
The Best Sources of Vitamin K2	*78*
Chapter 7	*Page 83*
The Cause of Toothaches	*83*
Foods and Lifestyles that Contribute to Toothaches	*85*
Chapter 8	*Page 89*

Weather and Toothaches	*89*
Solar Weather and Toothaches	*89*
Local Weather and Toothaches	*92*
A Dropping Dew Point Leads to Better Health	*93*

Chapter 9	*Page 97*
My Personal Experiences of 8 Years of Natural Healing of Toothaches	*97*

Chapter 10	*Page 100*
How to Properly Perform Oil Pulling	*100*
The Miracle of the Sunflower and how it Restores Hormone Levels Naturally	*101*

Chapter 11	*Page 106*
Actions You Can Take to Immediately Relieve a Toothache	*106*
In Case of Severe Tooth Pain	*111*

The Complete Guide to Natural Toothache Remedies and Re-mineralization

Why Cinnamon is More Effective than Clove in Reducing or Eliminating Toothache. The Scientific Evidence — *114*

Herbs and Compresses for Immediate Pain Relief — *115*

Using Ormus to help Relieve a Toothache — *116*

Chapter 12 — *Page 118*

Using Hydrogen Peroxide for Dental Hygiene and Health — *118*

Herbs for Mouth Rinses — *119*

How to Make Your Own Natural Breath Freshener — *119*

Chapter 13 — *Page 121*

Proven Techniques and Methods that Heal Dental Abscesses — *121*

How Gum Disease Increases Your Chances of a Stroke — *121*

How to use Niacin (vitamin B3) to Heal an Abscess	*123*
Using a Ginger and Mustard Footbath for Pain Relief	*126*
How to Use Golden Seal and Myrrh	*127*
Edible Bentonite Clay and Mineral Rich French Green Clay	*131*
Rapid Toxin Removal	*133*
A Formula For Relief of Inflamed Gums	*134*

Chapter 14	*Page 135*
Methods to Fight Infection and Boost the Immune System while Alleviating Toothache	*135*
Boosting Your Immune System	*116*

Chapter 15	*Page 138*
Foods for Healthy Teeth	*138*

The Complete Guide to Natural Toothache Remedies and Re-mineralization

Chapter 16 — *Page 139*

Cell Salts Known to Relieve Toothache — *139*

Chapter 17 — *Page 142*

Use the Power of Your Mind to Heal a Toothache — *142*

The Connection Between Stress and Toothaches — *143*

How Stress can Bring on a Toothache — *144*

Chapter 18 — *Page 146*

Natural Herbs for Gums with Inflammation and Bleeding Gums — *146*

Use Vitamin C in Grapefruit to Stop Bleeding Gums — *147*

Herbs for Healthy Gums — *149*

Quick Methods that Stop Bleeding Gums — *150*

*Herbs for Relief of
Periodontal Disease* — *150*

Chapter 19 — *Page 151*

*The Complete Master Herbal
List for Alleviating toothaches* — *151*

Chapter 20 — *Page 163*

*Understanding How Teeth
Remineralize Themselves* — *163*

Chapter 21 — *Page 167*

*Natural Cavity Repair Simply
Explained* — *167*

*How Amino Acids Help
Reverse Cavities* — *171*

The Miracle of Carnosine — *172*

Chapter 22 — *Page 176*

*Reviews of the best
Toothpastes that
Strengthen Tooth Enamel
and Re-mineralize Teeth* — *176*

The Complete Guide to Natural Toothache Remedies and Re-mineralization

How to Use
Remineralization Gels — *182*

All Natural Toothpastes
And Powders — *183*

Chapter 23 — *Page 185*

Nine 100% All Natural
Sugar Substitutes — *185*

Chapter 24 — *Page 191*

A Simple Diet Plan for
Dental Health — *191*

An Overall Summary of
the Nutrients that Create
Strong and Healthy Teeth — *192*

How to Use Grape
Seed Extract — *194*

Chapter 25 — *Page 196*

Herbal Mouth Ulcer and
Canker Sore Remedies — *196*

A Remedy for Canker Sores
and Dry Mouth — *197*

How To Make Your Own
Canker And Mouth Ulcer Salve   *197*

Chapter 26   *Page 198*

Jakob Lorber's Second
Sun Remedy   *198*

Chapter 27   *Page 204*

The Calcium to Phosphorous
Ratios of Foods   *204*

Chapter 28   *Page 207*

The Calcium to Phosphorous
Ratios of Fruits   *207*

Chapter 29   *Page 209*

The Oxalic acid Levels of
Foods   *209*

Chapter 30   *Page 211*

The Calcium Levels of
Vegetables   *211*

The Complete Guide to Natural Toothache Remedies and Re-mineralization

Chapter 31 — *Page 213*

The Calcium Levels of Fruit — *213*

Chapter 32 — *Page 215*

Levels of Vitamin C per 100 grams in Vegetables — *215*

Chapter 33 — *Page 217*

Vitamin C Levels per 100 grams in Fruit — *217*

Chapter 34 — *Page 219*

How to Make Your Own Zeolite Deotx Formula — *219*

Quoted Scientific References — *223*

Index: — *236*

Scott Rauvers

Testimonials from Readers of The Complete Guide to Natural Toothache Remedies and Re-mineralization

"Before reading The Complete Guide to Natural Toothache Remedies and Re-mineralization I had grown up believing in the authoritative care of dentists. They made me feel like a failure for having bad teeth. They treated me like cavities were a personal insult on the dental profession. After reading your book and applying the techniques, I no longer visit the dentist. Thank you for treating me like a person!"
-Erik

"This book is great! It empowered me and actually gave me more energy after using the techniques and herbs. I actually enjoy doing some of the exercises such as oil pulling and the mouth rinses because I feel great afterwards. By having this amazing book, I know I am truly being taken care of by someone who knows what he's talking about!"
-Debbie

"I had never had a cavity in my life until very recently. A friend of mine gave me his copy of The Complete Guide to Natural Toothache Remedies and Re-mineralization to read. After applying a few of the remedies provided, upon my return to the dentist, he was surprised to find my abscessed tooth had healed itself and that I no longer needed a root canal"
-Jeff

ACKNOWLEDGMENTS

Thank you to all the master herbalists and dentists who shared their toothache remedies with me.

Special thanks goes to Dr. Weston Price a fearless Pioneer of non-invasive methods to heal teeth.

Introduction

Haven't you ever wished you could have all the very best Ayurvedic, European and Traditional Chinese herbal remedies and scientifically proven tooth and gum healing remedies all in a convenient book?

You are holding in your hands the result of 5 years of research and writing, including feedback from readers of my website, the best natural remedies for healing toothache, gum disease and tooth abscesses.

This dream is now a reality. You won't find any other book that covers such a broad range of healing methods including herbal mouth rinses, and proven techniques to keep your teeth and gums free of pain and decay.

Best of all you no longer have to believe what your authoritarian dentist tells you. Unlike some books that fail to cite references backing up their claims, this book lists full references and the original scientifically published papers behind each claim made, allowing you, the reader to look up and confirm the validity of the information in this book for yourself.

How Mercury Damages the Body

There are many people who have concerns about having mercury used for their fillings. The mercury used in dental fillings is composed of dental amalgam.

What is Dental Amalgam?

Dental amalgam is composed of a 50/50 mixture of liquid mercury which is mixed with a powdered metal alloy of silver, copper and tin. When it is mixed it starts to form into a pliable putty-like substance that will harden.

In December 2010, the U.S. Food and Drug Administration warned against the use of using amalgam in vulnerable populations (the very old, very young and the pregnant). Pediatric Neurologist Dr. Suresh Kotagal testified at the FDA hearing "*there is no place for mercury in children.*" [1]

Developed Countries that have Banned the Use of Mercury Fillings

The European Union recently passed a resolution for all nations under the European Union to "*start restricting or prohibiting the use of amalgams as dental fillings.*" [2] [2a]

In 1987 the Public Health Office of Germany recommended against using amalgam in pregnant women, children, and people with kidney disease.

In July 1, 1995 Sweden ceased allowing amalgam to be used in patients under the age of twenty and banned it altogether in 1997.

In 1996, the Canadian Department of Health directed its dentists to cease using amalgam fillings altogether in children, pregnant women, and people with impaired kidney function. [3]

Early exposure to even low doses of mercury in women who are pregnant and breastfeeding have shown it causes an increased risk in having children with a lower intelligence. [4] This is because amalgam crosses the placenta and accumulates in unborn babies.

Why You Can Enjoy Better Health Using the Holistic Approach

Conventional dental treatments avoid the holistic approach altogether because it is not standard curriculum for students studying dentistry. The Complete Guide to Natural Toothache Remedies and Re-mineralization has sorted through all the confusion and misinformation, choosing only the best tried and proven holistic methods that work. The end result is a simple reference that can be accessed at your convenience. The beauty of this book is all 3 mainstream holistic treatments, Ayurvedic, Traditional Chinese and European are all brought together in one complete volume. This book includes the pioneering research done by Dr. Weston Price and Melvin Page presenting the facts and methods proven to work obtained from their research and scientific studies.

Prevention of cavities and treatment is so much more less painful and much less expensive than waiting until extensive tooth decay causes unsightly damaged teeth. Bad eating habits and digestion increases your chance of cavities, from unwanted plaque build-up on your teeth. If you have adequate amounts of stomach acid to digest the food you are eating, your plaque build-up will be substantially reduced.

The Complete Guide to Natural Toothache Remedies and Re-mineralization is a book you'll want to hand down to your grand kids generation after generation. Simple and quick protocols are presented in a clear straightforward manner for preventing cavities and remineralizing teeth. The beneficial side effects of using these proven holistic methods includes increased vitality and vibrancy due to restored hormone levels and the fresh intake of vitamins and minerals.

You may be surprised to learn that many of the most effective foods and spices that relieve toothache may already be in your kitchen cupboard. Clove for example is a powerful natural pain killer for toothache, and hydrogen peroxide mixed with water between 3% and 4% concentration is a powerful way to kill bad bacteria in the mouth that causes toothache.

In a genetic study of ancient dental plaque, researchers discovered that early man had at most 14% of their teeth covered in cavities and some showed almost no cavities at all.

Why Your Dentist Won't Share These Secrets With You

Many of these methods to highly educated people seem unorthodox and "messy". The fact is the further technology in medicine advances, the more science will reach the conclusion that nature provides the core principal ingredients needed for healing. I highly respect the Dental industry as they are very professional and can do amazing things with teeth and gums. They are miracle workers at taking care of the short term problem. However when it comes to long term dental health such as prevention which includes the diet, I believe that many of them ignore this area altogether, as Dental School never taught them the long term prevention techniques and foods that prevent cavities or the proper foods and procedures that re-mineralize teeth. This information is then passed on down to their patients, making the insurance companies very happy. Also cavities are healed with machines and mechanical devices and some companies making these machines do a pretty good business from selling them to dentists. Personally, I prefer the holistic organic methods any day.

An interesting note, as you may have seen so far, or will see later in this book, is that foods and herbs that contribute to perfect dental health also have significant anti-aging and cancer prevention traits. Maltitol, for example, which re-mineralizes teeth, has shown to be one of the most powerful foods for fly longevity experiments. Fruit Fly experiments showed 100 percent of the fruit flies surviving 18 days when fed Maltitol [4a]. The average life of a fruit fly is between 40 to 50 days. So with a 100% survival rate at 18 days being fed Maltitol is a pretty good survival rate. Longevity nutrition is hardly something clinically industrialized medicine today wants to promote.

Re-calcification of severe cavities is not only possible, but becoming more commonplace as more and more of this knowledge is revealed. Awareness of these non-painful methods will continue to grow, as people become more aware that using unnecessary resources only continues to destroy our planet and its health.

A Special Message To Dentists

From my experience over the years of talking to you, the dentist, in person, I have found many of you open to the methods that I have mentioned in this book. However, when it comes to long term dental health, I believe that many of you are uneducated, as Dental School never taught you the long term prevention foods, techniques and methods that help prevent cavities, or can suppress a toothache or are even aware of the natural methods proven to re-mineralize cavities. I believe a lot of this confusion comes from your insurance companies, who are happy keeping your patients in the dark about alternative methods of dental health and prevention.

When You, the Reader Should See A Dentist

A continuing toothache is the sign of something much more serious. So you should get to a dentist as soon as possible. However before you do, use the tips and techniques titled in the section of this book: "<u>Actions to Take Immediately if you Have a Toothache</u>" and you may just save a trip to the dentist. Pay particular attention to the section on abscesses as there are some great methods to help reduce the pain from them.

The Complete Guide to Natural Toothache
Remedies and Re-mineralization

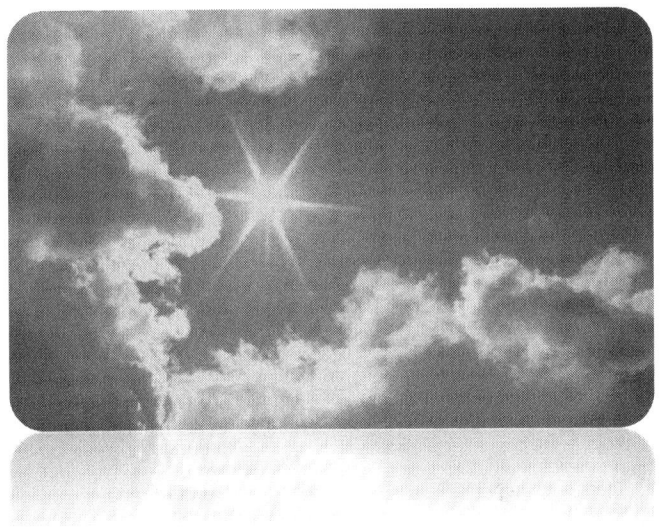

Scott Rauvers

Chapter 1

My Personal Story

Like some of you reading this, when I was younger I had healthy teeth, but as I approached a later age, I started to have teeth and gum problems. I wanted to share with readers what worked for me, as well as some of the best proven herbal toothache remedies that have helped thousands over the years, including the ancient time proven herbal remedies used for centuries.

This book has been designed to be kept short, simple and factual, numbering approximately 200 pages. The fact is the majority of dental visits for people with serious toothache don't require a root canal.

As more and more people are learning new and non-invasive ways to look after their teeth, Dentists are becoming more and more scared due to the shrinking lack of "*customers*" and are trying to find new and clever ways to keep people "*in the chair*". The fact is only your fear will keep you in the dentist's chair, because thousands of people each month are discovering that there are ways to avoid getting fillings, helping to re-calcify their teeth and avoid unnecessary root canals. For example in April 2014, health guru Dr. Mercola wrote an excellent article titled *"Why and How to Say No to an Unnecessary Root Canal Procedure"*. In the article he explains the clear lack of awareness people have about alternatives to root canals. Let's continue with my own story. I grew up in Australia, one of the best countries with excellent dental hygiene, with our school receiving half yearly visits from a travelling dentist who would keep our teeth clean and healthy, as well as give us fluoridation treatments. I never had any major cavity problems, until middle age. It was at this time I had my first root canal. This cost me an out of pocket expense of approximately $3,000. I had also had on and off cavities filled for the 7 years prior to this, including one filling that was improperly filled in and cracked my tooth 9 years later while I was eating. Anyway, it was only after the Internet arrived and the information matured enough, with feedback from others and good books on the topic, that I discovered that I could have excellent dental health, without root canals or painful gums and teeth. So after using many of the techniques and refining them further, I discovered that not only did they work, but I was able to eat about 5 to 8 bars of chocolate a week without any tooth problems.

After speaking in person with numerous dentists over the years and sharing these secrets with them, I have learned that there may be small "holes" in the teeth, but they will not cause excessive cavities if the right procedures and methods are taken. I have had a chipped tooth for over 3 years now that had the left part of my right gum exposed. By using these methods I am about to share in this book, I have never ever had any reoccurring decay, pain or cavities appear using them. I have used these maintenance and teeth rebuilding methods described in this book for the past 7 years without any problems.

Natural Tooth Repair Studies Performed by Dr. Weston Price

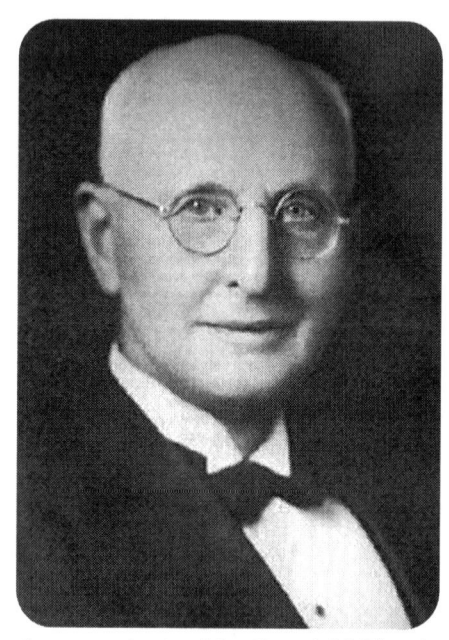

Dr. Weston A. Price, a Cleveland dentist, (*Born: September 6, 1870, Canada. Died: January 23, 1948*) demonstrated in the 1900's that native tribes who ate their traditional diet had almost zero cavities. And many of them were almost 100 percent free of tooth decay. These people did not use toothbrushes, floss or toothpaste. However when the tribal populations were introduced to sugar and foods high in white flour, their perfect teeth rapidly deteriorated. This proves an important link that nutrition is linked to the health of your teeth. Dr. Weston A. Price's book titled: *Nutrition and Physical Degeneration* is still a popular classic today, almost 100 years after its publication.

The book begins with research showing that the South African Bantu, when first visited by Dr. Price, had a low prevalence of tooth decay. This was because their diet was high in unrefined carbohydrate foods. Their decay rate increased rapidly as modern foods such as white flour and refined sugar was introduced into their diets.

Dr. Weston Price also documented the dramatic protective effect of cod liver oil (Vitamins A and D) and butter oil (Vitamins A and K2) against tooth decay. He used a combination of high-vitamin cod liver oil and high-vitamin butter oil to heal cavities, reduce oral bacteria counts, and cure numerous other afflictions in his patients. Dr. Price used extracts from grass-fed butter in combination with high vitamin cod liver oil to prevent and reverse dental cavities in many of his dental patients.

Butter contains numerous beneficial microbes that keep the teeth and gums healthy. Cod Liver Oil, Raw Organic Butter, Canola Oil and Sunflower Oil are fatty acid oils with long chains. Butter has large amounts of butyric acid, and is a potent antimicrobial and antifungal substance. Butter also contains conjugated linoleic acid (CLA) which gives excellent protection against cancer.

Why Vegetarians Get more Cavities

Dr. Price wrote in his book Nutrition and Physical Degeneration that vegetarian cultures had tooth decay at higher rates than those who ate meat. This was concluded after spending 10 years travelling around the world studying tooth decay in different cultures.

Because Dr. Price concluded that vegetarians are more prone to cavities, I found this to be true. As a matter of fact I had my first root canal done a few years after becoming vegetarian, as well as experiencing more toothaches than usual. However after adding carnosine to my diet, I have noticed that all toothaches ceased, and I was able to eat large amounts of chocolate, still without any cavities or toothaches. I attribute this to the carnosine. Meat happens to be high in the substance carnosine, especially the meat of chicken breast. A beneficial side effect of consuming carnosine is added energy. So by taking carnosine I am able to get all the benefits of meat without the problems or negative karma associated with heavy meat consumption.

What is Vitamin K2?

Vitamin K2 is the substance that makes the vitamin A and vitamin D dependent proteins come to life. While vitamins A and D act as signaling molecules, telling cells to make certain proteins, Vitamin K2 activates these proteins by conferring upon them the physical ability to bind calcium. In some cases these proteins directly coordinate the movement or organization of calcium themselves; in other cases the calcium acts as a glue to hold the protein in a certain shape. In all such cases, the proteins are only functional once they have been activated by vitamin K.

Vitamin K works with vitamin D to prevent bone loss and build new bone. To be absorbed properly, Vitamin K must be consumed with a fat such as Omega 3 or Omega 6 oils. Flaxseed is especially high in this.

Vitamin K2 is found in the highest levels in Natto. Natto is a type of fermented soybean often served on rice. When you eat it, it 'stretches' like spaghetti, so you have to wrap it around your fork. The best forms of K2 are found almost exclusively in fermented foods.

Food Sources of K2 from highest to

lowest: Parsley (Parsley is super high in Vitamin K, which the body makes into K2), Natto, Goose Liver Paste, Hard Cheeses and Soft Cheeses.

Additional sources of K2 include: Oregano, Cloves, Brussels sprouts, Parsley, Swiss Chard (raw), Watercress, Kale, Spinach, Beets, Collards and Chlorophyll.

Dairy products rich in this vitamin include egg whites, curd cheeses, butter and whole and low-fat milk.

Vitamin K2 Synergists: Cod Liver Oil (fermented Cod Liver Oil works best) & Butter Oil (100% grass-fed, unsalted cultured butter is the best), Vitamins A and D.

Vitamin K2 is best absorbed into the body with Cod Liver Oil and Organic Butter. It can also be taken with Coconut Oil & Palm Oil. The close cousin to K2, Vitamin K, also can be used for dental health. It works with vitamin D to prevent bone loss and build new bone. Alfalfa is also high in

Vitamin K.

A good all purpose food that naturally contains high amounts of Vitamin K is Chlorophyll. Chlorophyll is rich in vitamin K and oxygenates human cells by helping to build red blood cells. Chlorophyll has been effective in halting tooth decay and gum infections, probably due to its high oxygen content. Chlorophyll is also used for treating inflammation, helping renew tissues and activating enzymes in the body to help produce Vitamin K. Chlorophyll can be found in the following foods: Spinach, Chard, Kale, Collard, Mustard, Alfalfa And Sea Vegetables. The highest levels are found in Spirulina, Chlorella and Blue Green Algae. Hydrogen Peroxide is the next substance that contains high amounts of oxygen.

Chapter 2

Simple and Effective Herbal Formulas for Teeth and Gums

In this chapter we have put together the best herbal formulas from all 3 world traditions spanning thousands of years. They are: Traditional Chinese Herbal Medicine, Homeopathic, European Herbal Formulas and Tinctures. We also include a section on North American Indian Remedies for Toothache. Let's begin with Rosemary Gladstar.

Rosemary Gladstar's Healing Mouthwash

Rosemary Gladstar is a master herbalist. She has been referred to as The Godmother of American Herbalism. Over 35 years ago in her shop named Rosemary's Garden in Sonoma County, California, she developed herbal formulas which have helped thousands over the years.

Here is her famous Healing Mouthwash:

3/4 cup water
1/4 cup vodka
40 drops calendula tincture
40 drops goldenseal tin tire
20 drops myrrh tincture
1 or 2 drops peppermint essential oil.

Combine the ingredients and seal in an airtight glass bottle. Use for inflamed gums or as a preventive mouthwash.

You will find that many of the herbs that help heal gums are astringent herbs. These astringent herbs help tighten and reduce inflammation.

The Jean Valnet Remedy

The famous French aromatherapy doctor Jean Valnet (shown on the next page), practiced aromatherapy for more than 30 years.

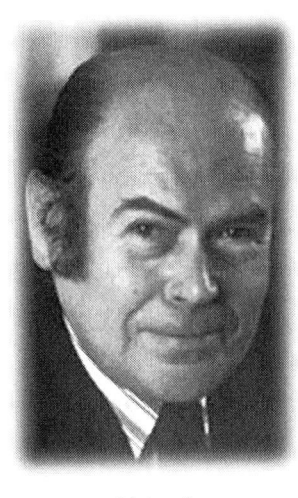

Jean prescribed the following formula for toothache:

1.8oz of arnica flowers
0.4oz of clove buds
0.4oz of cinnamon
0.4 oz of Ginger root
3.5oz ounces of anise seeds
34oz of Vodka.

Because these are such strong astringent herbs, be sure to where possible use 100 proof vodka or similar. It takes a strong alcohol to dissolve these strong herbs. To prepare:

Place the herbs into the alcohol for 8 to 12 days.

After 8 to 12 days strain through a coffee filter and store in a glass airtight bottle out of direct sunlight and keep away from heat.

To use, take 1 teaspoon of the infusion in half a glass of warm water mixed with 1 teaspoon of raw honey that is dissolved in 4 ounces of warm water. Rinse the mouth out 2 to 3 times a day after eating. After rinsing, spit out the solution. Let's move onto a American herbal remedy.

A Preventive Health Mouth Wash

This is a standard mouth wash to create healthy teeth and gums. Mix the following herbs and essential oils together.

1oz of goldenseal
1/2oz of myrrh
2 drops peppermint essential oil
2 drops cinnamon essential oil

Begin by heating the goldenseal and myrrh in water just before it gets boiling. After the water has cooled, add the peppermint and cinnamon. Store the remainder of the liquid in a glass airtight bottle out of direct sunlight and keep away from heat.

Jerthro Kloss Gum Healer and Mouth Rinse

Gather the following herbs:
2oz myth
1oz goldenseal
0.5oz cayenne

Mix the above into a 1 quart glass jar with 100 proof alcohol with plastic lining the inside lid. Next shake each day for between 7 and 10 days. After 10 days strain through a coffee filter and store in a glass airtight bottle out of direct sunlight and keep away from heat.

Use the above in a poultice. This formula also has multipurpose uses. For example it has been found to be of benefit when used for Sunburns, Wounds, Bruises, Sprains, Scalds, Burns, and Pyorrhea of the Gums.

If you don't have 100 proof or better alcohol, than use the strongest alcohol possible. You can learn more about how to make your own tinctures in my book; How to Make Tinctures, Extracts, Flower Essences and Homeopathic Remedies.

An Ancient Chinese Herbal Remedy for Toothache

Mix the following herbs together in even amounts and make into a tincture. Anemone Cernua, Fo Ti (He Shou Wu), Angelica Anomala, Selenium Monnieri, Asarum Sieboldii, Quercus (also used to heal gingivitis) and Dentata. Once your tincture is made, add between 8 and 15 drops to a cup of warm water and use as a mouth rinse.

Michael Moore's Tooth Powder

Michael Moore was a master herbalist and practitioner of American Herbalism during the second half of the 20th century. With

The Complete Guide to Natural Toothache Remedies and Re-mineralization

40+ years experience, his written works made him one of the leading master herbalists in America.

You can find over 100 of Michael's herbal formulas by doing an Internet search for the term: HERBAL FORMULAS FOR CLINIC AND HOME or by visiting the following website at the address below:
http://www.swsbm.com/ManualsMM/Formulary2.txt

When mixing the herbs in Michael's formula shown below, be sure to grind them as finely as possible. If the air happens to be extra dry such as during summer, be sure to wear a mask. The key is that the more fine you can grind up the powder, than the better it is able to get in between the teeth, where it can feed the good bacteria and destroy the bad bacteria. To begin, gather the following herbs:

12 oz Arrowroot
4oz orris root
1oz baking soda
1oz licorice root

1oz myrrh
1oz cloves
1oz cinnamon
1oz Yerba mansa
20 drops peppermint essential oil
10 drops wintergreen essential oil

After thoroughly mixing all of the above, briefly blend. Blend no more than one half cup at a time. Use as a mouth rinse or apply as a poultice, placed next to the gum line closest to the toothache.

Suitable Replacements:

Baking soda can be substituted for baking powder.
Nutmeg can be substituted for cinnamon.
5 drops clove can be substituted for wintergreen and peppermint.
You can also add some fine pepper for extra "zing".

Jared's Tooth Powder

Jared Tropple, a Master Herbalist for more than 8 years, recommends the following formula for toothache relief.

Orris Root Powder 4 ounces
Arrowroot 4 ounces
Myrrh Gum 2 ounces
Licorice Root 1.5 ounces
White Oak Bark 1.5 ounces
Golden Seal Root 1 ounce
Bistort Root 1 ounce
Peppermint Oil 1/2 teaspoon

After powdering all the herbs into a fine powder, mix them thoroughly with the Peppermint Oil. Place near gum where toothache is present for immediate relief.

Jakob Lorber's Tooth Remedy Powder

Jakob Lorber's caries powder is made from plum tree ash that has been exposed to the light of the sun. It is taken with sunned plum schnaps and applied to the toothache twice daily for 3 days. It is reputed to make carious lesions in the teeth vanish. Some people have mixed the plum tree ashes and schnaps with non-abrasive natural toothpaste. In a German website forum devoted to users of Jakob Lorber's Tooth Powder, users state that it improved the dental health of low income women in Romania who had a diet of poor nutrition. The powder can also be mixed with toothpaste. Below is the original text taken from his book titled: The Healing Power of Sunlight, published in 1851. You can also read the entire book online at: www.franky1.com/Sun.pdf .

Here is the text as follows:
In addition to what I have already told you, I will give you some further medications, prepared through the rays of the sun, which are to be used externally rather than internally and which you may call sympathetic sunray remedies. Take branches, including the bark, of a plum tree and burn them to ashes. It would be best if you had a burning glass or a concave mirror in order to burn, in its focus, the plum tree wood, which would, of course, have to be cut into small chips, to ashes. The ashes must then be exposed to the rays of the sun for 5 to 8

days, and that in a dark vessel rather than a light one. After the ashes have thus been prepared through the rays of the sun they must, like the other medications, be carefully protected from the external air in a dry little bottle. Someone with a decayed tooth can then take 5 to 8 grains of it, on a not too hard toothbrush which, prior to that, has to be dipped in sunned plum spirits. With this ash, the decayed tooth has to be brushed for 3 days in the mornings and evenings and the decay will be healed and the tooth, finally, completely restored. Similar ashes may be prepared also from the stalks of sage which have been treated in the same way, except that the toothbrush is not dipped in plum spirits, but in spirits of wine of approximately 40%, after this has been impregnated with etheric oils of sage. To impregnate the spirits of wine with the etheric oils of sage, add 10 drops of this oil to 1/8 of a pint, the little bottle is plugged up, the contents shaken and then exposed to the rays of the sun for 5-8 days. Then the bottle is wrapped in dark paper and stored in a dry place.

Towards the end of this book you can find another sun remedy by Jakob.

Ayurvedic Methods for Healing Toothache

In the Eastern Indian tradition of Ayurvedic healing, a toothache is caused by the body being overly acidic. Other conditions include: receding gums, and being sensitive to heat. In the case of receding gums, the nerves near the teeth become sensitive to cold or heat. If a person is sensitive to cold, they may have receding gums, if they are sensitive to heat, this indicates signs of infection.

If the person has high acid, they will be susceptible to heartburn, and acid indigestion. This can be controlled by taking up a pitta soothing diet which rebalances digestion, metabolism, and energy production. This includes avoiding spicy foods, fermented foods such as pickles and citrus fruits. You can use natural edible camphor (but not the synthetic kind because it is toxic) placed next to the tooth and allow the saliva to mix with the camphor to relieve the pain. Ayurvedic healing also recommends the herb; Pellitory of the Wall for treating paralysis, epilepsy and as an overall health tonic. It has traditionally been used for restoring to the kidneys and the bladder.

Time Tested Chinese Herbal Remedies for Toothache

The Rehmannia Six Combination (Liu wei di huang wan)

An old favorite in use for many years, this formula has multiple uses. Other uses of Rehmannia 6 include: anemia (tired blood), diabetes, fever, weakened bones (osteoporosis), and allergies. You can buy many prepared formulas of Rehmannia 6 from reputable online merchants.

To make this combination yourself gather the following herbs:

20-30 gms of prepared Rehmannia (Rehmannia glutinosa) (Chinse Name: Shu Di Huang)

10-15 gms of Cornus (Cornus officinalis) (Chinese Name: Shan Zhu Yu)

10-15 gms of Dioscorea (Dioscorea opposita) (Chinese Name: Shan Yao)

9-12 gms of Water Plantain (Alisma plantago-aquatica) (Chinese Name: Ze Xie)

6-9 gms of Moutan Peony (Paeonia suffruticosa) (Chinese Name: Mu Dan Pi)

9-12 gms of Poria (Poria cocos) (Chinese Name: Fu Ling)

Make into a tincture and place on tooth. You can also take between 5 and 8 drops with a glass of water for internal use.

The Niu Huang Jie Du Pian Formula

Niu Huang Jie Du Pian was first listed in "Differentiation Standards" a Volume on Gynecology and Pediatrics" (Bian Zheng Zhun Sheng Fu Yu Ji). This volume dates back to the Ming Dynasty, (*1368 to 1644AD*), so it has proven itself for hundreds of years. It helps heal infections of mouth and tongue ulcers. In traditional Chinese medicine it can be used to treat constipation caused by excessive heat that is not associated with a Yin deficiency. It can also be used for earaches, sore throats, conjunctivitis, and headaches associated with strong fire (Fire is a Chinese Medicine Term related to the 4 treatment elements) so it is especially good for treating the upper part of the body. It can also be used for symptoms of aversion to wind, cough, headache, thirst and throat pain. Also constipation caused by excess heat (not Deficient Yin type of constipation). Additional uses include: pneumonia, pharyngitis, otitis media, fever, common cold, flu, acute bronchitis, parotitis, measles, tonsilitis.

It can also be applied directly to the skin to remove boils, sores, carbuncles and similar skin inflections. Take this formula with plenty of water as it will go to work detoxing your body. Like the Rehammnia 6 formula, it can be purchased in tablet form from a reputable merchant. It can also be made into a tincture and taken internally by adding between 5 and 10 drops at a time to a warm cup of water. Its main power comes from fighting inflammation, especially inflammation in the upper part of the body. Additional uses include relief of the following: Headache, vertigo, sore throat, gastric fever, mouth pimples, tongue ulcers, dry throat or mouth, bleeding gums, acute ophthalmia, acute dysphasia, mumps, earache, toothache, children's fever, anorexia, nausea. In Amazon.com when purchased in tablet, form it averages between 4.5 and 5 stars, very high ratings for a Chinese herbal medicine, so it has a good review rating making it highly effective.

The Complete Guide to Natural Toothache Remedies and Re-mineralization

Directions:

If you don't want to make a tincture of Niu Huang Jie Du Pian, you can purchase it in tablet form from a reputable online merchant. To use, take 2 tablets twice daily. Once in the morning and again in the evening with warm water. The children's dose is to be reduced by half. In more severe cases, especially with toothache, take 2 tablets, 3 or 4 times a day with lots of water.

You can also use the formula below to make your own tincture.

Chinese Name -- Common Name -- Latin Name -- Milligrams

Jin Yin Hua - Honeysuckle Flower, Flos Lonicerae - 360

Lian Qiao - Forsythia Fruit, Fructus Forsythiae - - 360

Niu Bang Zi - Arctium Fruit, Fructus Arctii Burdock Fruit - 215

Jie Geng - Platycodon Root, Balloon Flower Root - 215

Dan Dou Chi - Fermented soybean, Semen

Sojae Preparatum – 215

Dan Zhu Ye – Lophatherum, Herba Lophatheri – 200

Bo He – Mentha, Herba Menthae, Chinese Mint – 145

Jing Jie – Schizonepeta Schizonepetae, Herba Seu Flos – 145

Gan Cao – Licorice Root Uralensis, Radix Glycyrrhizae– 145

The Chinese herb Baizhi

The Chinese herb Baizhi (common name Angelica) can be used for severe tooth abscesses. It works also to relieve headache.

The Chinese herb Xuchangqing

The next Chinese herb called Xuchangqing also called the Root Of Paniculate Swallowwort (scientific name: cynanchum paniculatum) relieves pain. It creates moisture and is also used for abdominal pain during menstruation and stomach ache. It can be toxic if used in high amounts. It is also effective in relieving cough. It exerts a warm energy and is used to relieve sputum and for antirheumatic pain.

Native American Toothache Remedies

California Poppy (Eschscholzia californica). Poppy has been used by Indians on the west coast for toothaches and earaches for hundreds of years.

Caltrop (Kallstroemia grandiflora). Native Americans chewed the leaves of this plant for toothache. A poultice of Caltrop is used for skin sores and bruises.

After placing the powdered root in warm water, it can be used as a wash for sore and tired eyes.

Yerba Buena (Satureja douglasii). The Costanoan Indians hold the leaves of Yerba in their mouth to treat toothaches. The leaves can also be heated in a microwave or over a warm fire and made into a poultice and placed on the outside jaw to treat toothache. This herb can also be made into a strong decoction and used for treating pinworms, as a carminative for colic, a blood purifier, a reliever of arthritic symptoms, a febrifuge, and as a general tonic and panacea. The leaves are also used to heal upset stomachs.

Plantain (Plantago major and P lanceolata). The Chippewa Indians used plantain leaves to draw out splinters from inflamed skin, and as vulnerary poultices. Plantain will staunch blood flow quickly, encouraging the rapid repair of tissue. It is commonly used in place of comfrey for mending broken bones. Plantain roots can be chewed or powdered and used for toothache.

Sweetgum (Liquidambar styraciflua). Native Americans applied the resin of Sweetgum directly to the cheek to ease toothache. The twigs of Sweetgum can be soaked in water or whiskey and chewed to clean the teeth. Sweetgum resin can be chewed and used as a tooth cleaner and for sweetening the breath. This is a multipurpose herb that can also be used for the following: treating fevers and wounds, herpes and skin inflammations.

Use Sweetgum resin for:

Treating boils, toothache and tuberculosis. It can also be made into incense, perfumery, soaps and as a strong natural adhesive. When chewed, sweetgum will relieve sore throats, coughs, asthma, cystitis, dysentery etc. When used externally it will help treat piles, sores, wounds, ringworm, scabies etc. The mildly astringent inner bark of Sweetgum has been used to treat diarrhea and childhood cholera.

Using Watermelon Rind for Toothache

This formula is hundreds of years old and has been documented by Ben Cao Hui Yan of the Ni Zhu-Mo, Ming dynasty (1368 - 1644 d. C.) in the Treasury of Words on the Materia Medica. The instructions state to *'burn dried watermelon rind until it turns to ash. Next place a tiny amount of ash on the gum line closet to the aching tooth."* Watermelon is also one of the top 10 anti-aging foods, having numerous health benefits. Because the melon cantaloupe is related to Watermelon, there are some people who have also used cantaloupe for toothaches. The instructions state to take about 6 grams of cantaloupe skin and after adding water, simmer gently. Next it is strained and used as a mouth rinse.

How to Make Herbs into Fine Powder

If you want to make really fine powder out of herbs, use a very fine metal tea strainer. Locate the one with the finest mesh. Next grind up the herbs in a mortar and pestle or coffee grinder as finely as you can. Next open a large plastic bag and place the open end of the bag over the edge of a table, securing one end with a weight. Next place the tea strainer over the plastic bag and empty the crushed herbs into the strainer. Next gently tap the side of the strainer over the top of the plastic bag onto a hard surface such as the corner of a table. This allows the crushed herbs to expel their powder through the strainer and into the plastic bag via gravity. Place the rough herbs back into the coffee grinder or mortar and pestle and repeat until you have a bag filled with extra fine herb powder. Be sure to wear a mask if the air is extra dry as the powder will get into your nasal areas.

Essential Oils and Herbs for Relief of Toothache

Out of all toothache healing remedies, essential oils are the most concentrated. That is why using only 1 to 3 drops are all that is necessary for instant relief.

Thyme

Use Thyme essential oil mixed with water to create a mouth wash or reduce inflammation.

Wintergreen

Use essential oil of Wintergreen by applying 1 drop directly on the aching tooth.

Oregano Essential Oil

Dilute 5 drops oregano essential oil to 25 drops of carrier oil such as jojoba oil and rub directly on the gum closest to the toothache.

Cypress oil

Cypress oil has haemostatic, astringent, antiseptic and vasoconstrictor properties making it great for bleeding gums.

Eucalyptus

A powerful natural anti-inflammatory, and natural antibacterial antiseptic. In a study titled "Chewing Gum Supplemented with Eucalyptus Extract May Improve Periodontal Health" which was published in the 2008 Journal of Periodontology, researchers concluded that the use of eucalyptus chewing gum promoted periodontal health.
View the study at:
www.ncbi.nlm.nih.gov/pubmed/18672986)

Cajuput

This essential oil has a sweet aroma and penetrates deeply into tissue. The species of Cajuput is closely related to tea tree oil. Dilute with Carrier oils and massage into sore or bleeding gums

Lavender

A beautiful calming aroma, believed to work best around full moons, Lavender enhances blood circulation and tissue formation.

Camomile oil

A powerful natural antiseptic and antibiotic. It helps fight inflammation. Camomile works best when combined with Tea Tree Oil. To use, make a mouth rinse consisting of between 3 and 4 drops of Camomile and 3 and 4 drops of Tea Tree Oil in 3 ounces of water and rinse mouth 3 times a day to ward off infection associated with receding gums.

Kombucha tea

Author Rosina Fasching has described in her book "Tea Fungus Kombucha: The Natural Remedy and its Significance in Cases of Cancer and Other Metabolic Diseases" that regular drinkers of Kombucha tea have strong healthy teeth. Like Roobios Tea, Kombucha is reputed to also contain natural fluoride. Some people freak out that anything with fluoride in it is bad for them. The fact is herbs and teas that contain natural fluoride contain it in such small amounts they actually do more good than harm. The fluoride amounts in drinking water and toothpaste contain thousands more Parts Per Million (PPM) fluoride than that contained in herbs. This is why drinkers of Roobios and Kombucha tea have healthier teeth.

Because teas help promote good bacteria in your stomach, it is best to rotate different types of teas every now and then. This creates a healthy balance so that the symbiotic culture of bacteria in your stomach does not get used to the same type of tea. Much like bacteria can become resistant to the same antibiotics, the symbiotic culture of bacteria that fights infection and gives your body immunity can actually become depleted over time if you keep drinking the same type of tea constantly. From my personal experience, I like to drink Roobios tea 2 days in a row, take a break than drink Passion flower tea for 1 day, than take a 2 day break and go back to Roobios Tea. You don't have to be strict on rotation, just vary your tea consumption routine enough so that intuitively you find the best plan that suits you.

There have also been studies done where the urine of individuals who had never consumed Kombucha before showed considerable traces of environmental toxins including benzene, cesium, lead and mercury after drinking Kombucha tea. This was even after the Kombucha tea had been tested for metallic contaminants. This means an added advantage of drinking Kombucha tea may be of benefit for those suffering from heavy metal toxicity.

How to use Eucalyptus Oil

To use for massaging into gums, mix eucalyptus essential oil with a carrier oil such as Jojoba, Grape seed or Almond oil than gently massage into the gums affected by periodontal disease.

Natural Tea Contains High Amounts of Fluoride

According to the USDA Nutrient Database, Tea contains between 1.15 and 3.93 ppm of fluoride with unsweetened instant tea powder containing a whopping 897.72 ppm. According to the paper on the following page titled: "USDA National Fluoride Database of Selected Beverages and Foods, Release 2", instant tea is the food with the highest levels of fluoride available. This is because in the world of herbs, some herbs, when they become dried into powder naturally increase their levels of nutrients. Dried Kale is one example. In the case of tea, the fluoride levels are off the charts.
http://www.ars.usda.gov/SP2UserFiles/Place/80400525/Data/Fluoride/F02.pdf

Other foods that naturally contain fluoride include: Cottage Cheese, Cheddar Cheese, Oats, Raisins, Cranberry Juice, Carbonated Tonic Water and Rye Bread.

From my personal experience, my diet is

high in Raisins and also during winter I eat more Cottage Cheese than usual. So these foods may also be assisting in strengthening tooth enamel.

Chapter 3

Keeping the Gums Healthy

In this chapter we are going to explore methods that you can use to ensure long term prevention of tooth decay and gum disease.

Healthy gums are gums that are strong, tight and a have a healthy pink color. Periodontal Disease is simply caused by a lack of healthy CQ10 levels in the body. Sardines, which are high in CQ10, also contain Omega 3 Oils, which are needed if the body is to effectively use CQ10. The good thing about sardines is that because they are such small fish, they have hardly any mercury poison like the larger fish do, so they are very safe to eat.

Supplements are also available, however for proper absorption into the body Omega 3 oils must accompany the CQ10. Other foods rich in CQ10 are raw peanuts, spinach and wheat germ. Fish are high in

CQ10, but the bigger the fish, the more mercury.

I have got great results eating sardines with sprouted flax or chia seeds. Chia and flax seeds are high in Omega 3 fatty acids. In fact, chia seeds contain more Omega-3s than salmon, gram for gram.

Black or Green Tea for Healthy Gums

In a study published in the Journal of Periodontology [5], 940 Japanese men aged between 49 and 59 who had gum (*periodontal*) disease which involved bleeding or receding gums drank a minimum of one cup of green tea each day. At the end of the study these men showed improvement in their receding gums including a reduction in their bleeding gums. The researchers concluded that the improvement was from the catechins in the green tea, which reduced inflammation resulting from bacteria in the mouth.

In a research study titled: "The Tea Catechin Epigallocatechin Gallate Suppresses Cariogenic Virulence Factors of Streptococcus mutans" [6] researchers Xin Xu,1,2 Xue D. Zhou,2 and Christine D. Wu1 and their team performed a study on the effects of catechins and polyphenols and tooth health. Their study stated catechins and polyphenols inhibited the growth of oral bacteria by killing the bad bacteria over a 48-hour incubation period.

The laboratory study concluded that polyphenols found in tea also killed three species of bacteria associated with bad breath for 48 hours and at concentrations ranging between 16 and 250 micrograms per milliliter. The polyphenols also reduced the growth of oral bacteria. What was more surprising was that at low concentrations of polyphenols (*between 2.5 and 25 micrograms per milliliter*), the polyphenols inhibited the enzyme that causes the formation of hydrogen sulfide, cutting its production by 30 percent.

The Role Hydrogen Sulfide plays in the

mouth is that it is emitted by tiny bacteria. This bacteria comes from a chemical reaction caused when the bacteria eat small particles that get wedged in-between the teeth. Hydrogen sulfide is the same compound that gives rotten eggs their characteristic smell.

Periodontal Disease, one of the more common forms of gum disease, is simply caused by a lack of adequate levels of CQ10 levels in the body.

In a scientific study titled: "Pilot Study Of Dietary Fatty Acid Supplementation In The Treatment Of Adult Periodontitis" [7] researchers used a combination of fish oil, eicosapentaenoic acid, and borage oil on volunteers suffering from periodontitis. The researchers concluded that the Borage Oil had beneficial effects reducing inflammation caused by people suffering from periodontal disease.

Oolong tea has also been shown to be a powerful cavity prevention tea.

Herbal Remedies for Healthy Gums

Tight gums are healthy gums. Tight gums help to prevent food borne particles from getting caught in between the teeth. I have found that my teeth are healthier when my gums are tight.

Rosemary. If your gums are "too tight", use rosemary. Just add a teaspoon or two to hot water, than cool. Next gargle and rinse your mouth out.

Willow. The main ingredient in willow is salicin, which has effects similar to aspirin. It is powerful for healing inflammation anywhere in the upper part of the body. You can chew on the willow herb directly, or apply topically to the tooth for pain relief. Oak can also be used. Willow and oak together in a poultice are good for toothache. Oak can also be combined with willow in equal parts to make an equally good and effective poultice.

Natural Methods That Tighten Gums

Below are three main techniques for tightening gums:

Oil Puling with Sunflower oil (*which we will cover more in-depth later on in this book*)

Drinking Cranberry Juice with Garlic

Eating Sardines

Myrrh powder has also been used with success to heal teeth and gums. One of the most effective natural remedies to tighten gums I have found is by placing freshly sliced garlic in cranberry juice. After just a few hours, you can really feel the gums of the teeth start to tighten up. This is because Cranberry has the highest antioxidant activity out of any berry as shown in a study titled: "Antioxidant and Antiproliferative Activities of Common Fruits." [8]

Fast Fact: Omega 3 fatty acids combined with resveratrol create a powerful anti-aging cocktail mix.

Foods rich in CQ10: Raw peanuts (*hint: If you sprout the raw peanuts you increase the resveratrol amounts in them substantially*), spinach and wheat germ. Fish are high in CQ10, but the bigger the fish, the more mercury.

Brushing teeth and gums with Ormus (*we will cover Ormus later on in this book*) has also been found to help. Grape Juice is highly alkaline, and if you swish your mouth with grape juice than swish or brush your teeth with Ormus it creates healthy teeth and gums.

Chapter 4

Herbs to Build Strong Teeth

Pau d Arco Bark. Besides being used as a poultice for toothache, it is also used as poultice for backaches.

Basil. Commonly used in mouthwashes, as it helps the gum tissues absorb the ingredients better.

Lavender and Tea Tree Oil. Add 3 drops Lavender to 2 drops tea tree oil and mix well. Place on gum line near tooth for relief.

Calamus (Acorus americanus). Make into a poultice and place next to gum line of toothache. Works well for extreme toothaches.

Calendula (Calendula officinalis). For thousands of years, tinctures of calendula blossoms have been used to bring relief to headaches, toothaches and tuberculosis, due to its ability to act upon the upper part of the body.

Carnosine (*not a herb, but an amino acid. It strengthens teeth*).

I have also had much success using a combination of Rooibos Tea and Pumpkin Seeds. This combination of pumpkin seeds and Roobios Tea is commonly used as a tea blend. Rooibos Tea has been used as a natural cavity prevention drink for many years by people in Africa. After drinking Roobios Tea, my teeth and gums are much more tighter and stronger. I have found taking the Roobios Tea and Pumpkin seeds combination works best right after oil pulling. What is interesting is Pumpkin Seeds have been shown to help balance hormones around the full moon. Could taking Roobios Tea around the full moon also have a similar hormone balancing effect? Further studies are needed to confirm this. You can also buy Pumpkin Rooibos Tea bags with the Rooibos tea and pumpkin seeds already combined in a convenient tea bag from Amazon.com

In a scientific study titled: "Anti-Oxidative Effects of Rooibos Tea (Aspalathus linearis) on Immobilization-Induced Oxidative Stress in Rat Brain", [37] researchers found that Roobios tea significantly lowered the body's stress levels by increasing its resistance to stress. Further research needs to be done on Roobios to see if it has a positive effect on hormones.

Natural Non-Invasive Methods that Strengthen Teeth

The best herbs that strengthen teeth are:

Alflafa. horsetail, nettle, oatstraw. From personal experience, I have had excellent results with Horsetail Tea and mixing ground up Horsetail herb with Spirulina in a 50/50 ratio and mixing it with plain greek yogurt.

Some herbs work best when combined together. Let's look at one combination.

The Complete Guide to Natural Toothache Remedies and Re-mineralization

To improve the condition of teeth, simmer one ounce of each the following in one pint of water for 25 minutes and take 1/2 cup 2 to 3 times daily. After 3 weeks stop for one week. This combination works especially well during wintertime.

1 part horsetail (rich in silica)
1 part oatstraw (rich in silica)
1 part kombu seaweed or kelp powder (rich in minerals)
1/2 part lobelia (promotes relaxation)

In a scientific study titled: "Effect of combined administration of vitamin D3 and vitamin K2 on bone mineral density of the lumbar spine in postmenopausal women with osteoporosis", [9] Researchers discovered that when Vitamin D3 was taken with Vitamin K2, it helped increase the absorption of Vitamin K into the body.

Because either too much Vitamin A or too much Vitamin D together can cause toxicity in the body, when they are both combined together in the right ratios and taken in large doses, it actually works the opposite. It is good for the body.

Professor I.G. Spiesman at the University of Illinois College of Medicine suggested that both vitamins A and D worked together to prevent infection because both these vitamins are necessary to prevent the common cold [28].

In 1941 he published his own findings concluding that massive doses of each vitamin taken separately often caused toxicity in the body, however when he studied massive doses of both vitamins taken together, it offered powerful protection against the common cold.

Researchers at Tuff's University conducted a similar study and also came to the same conclusion as Professor Spiesman [11]. Research has also shown that vitamins A and D work together with vitamin K to activate proteins that support mineralization of bones and teeth as published in a study conducted by Dr. Price [12].

Foods that are high in Vitamin A include Spinach and Cod Liver Oil. So a healthy toothache recovery meal would be Natto and Spinach with Cod Liver Oil Capsules.

The Best Tree Bark for Strong Teeth

Chew any of the barks for strong and healthy teeth:

Bay, Beech, Birch, Dogwood, Fir, Eucalyptus, Juniper, Maple, Neem, Oak Pine, Poplar And Sumac.

Using Parsley For Re-Strengthening Loose Teeth

Drink 3 cups of parsley leaf daily. Eat raw carrots with celery for strong gums. Carrots and celery are good sources of beta carotene which your body needs to create vitamin A. Vitamin A is a nutrient essential for building strong teeth.

The Best Teas for Healthy Teeth and Gums

Over the years I have discovered that drinking Rooibos tea has an extremely beneficial effect on tightening my gums, and helping keep my teeth strong. I believe this comes from Rooibos' tea's ability to reduce or heal inflammation, especially inflammation at the cellular level. In a Japanese Study conducted using Roobios tea, researchers concluded that Rooibos tea may prevent DNA damage and inflammation due to its anti-oxidant activity. The study also concluded that due to the gentle effects of Roobios tea, it is safe for young children. [13] Roobios tea is also caffeine free.

Methods to Tighten Gums

When gums are tight, they are not only healthy, but they help to prevent food borne particles from getting caught in between the teeth.

As we covered earlier, swishing the mouth with Hydrogen Peroxide also helps tighten the teeth and gums. So we can see that the natural long term solutions to preventing tooth decay and gum disease are far ahead of the "brush 3 times per day" ideology.

Natural Herbs for Oral Hygiene and Healthy Teeth

BloodRoot. This herb is one of the more commonly used herbs for dental health because it contains Sanguinarine, which is a powerful natural anti-plaque substance that fights tooth decay and gum disease. Some companies are now using it with mouthwashes and toothpastes.

Using Coconut Oil to Dissolve Plaque

When coconut oil and tea tree are combined they create a powerful healing

effect. Some people have successfully used this combination on their face as a successful method to fight acne. To fight plaque and strengthen gums;
Take 1/8 oz of coconut oil and add 8 drops oil of myrrh, 8 drops tea tree oil and 2 drops peppermint oil. Shake well and massage a few drops into gums.

Neem. Sticks of Neem can be chewed between the teeth to produce beneficial bacteria in the mouth that fights tooth infection. Neem also makes a powerful natural garden insect repellent. It is one of the best non-chemical herbal pesticides available. This proves that Neem has powerful properties that kill and repel bad bacteria.

Chapter 5

How Diet and Sugar Relate to Dental Health

At various times our bodies become stressed and the hormones imbalanced and we turn to sugary foods for comfort. The effects of sugar on the body are only temporary. This gives anyone the opportunity to stay off sugar for just 7 days and see a significant improvement in their teeth and gums.

A Simple Sugar Detox Plan

When the body is under excessive stress, or becomes overly laden with industrial pollutants or toxins, sugar suppresses the ability of the body to effectively repair itself.

Once the body has been flushed free of sugar, either by taking moderate amounts of grapefruit or parsley and drinking lots of purified or spring water, the sugar cravings cease. If one abstains from chocolate for 5 to 10 days and takes plenty of vitamins C and D, when one returns to eating chocolate, it may no longer taste as it once did. The "spark" has died. I believe the reason for this is because as the body is flushed of sugar it becomes more alkaline, which alters the sensations and experiences of sugar. This proves sugar cravings are part physical with a minor part of the cravings being mental, such as using sugar as a comfort food during times of stress or minor depression.

My Experience of Abstaining From Sugar

After not eating sugar for 7 days I have found the following;

Ability to think more clearly
More longer term energy. This is because there is no "sugar crash".

Are able to think and reason much more quickly

My immune system is stronger and healthier

The food I eat absorbs more nutrients

I feel mentally stronger

I want to eat healthier foods

I don't feel as if there are "missing nutrients" in my diet

My skin is not as dry

Simply put, sugar, the number 1 tooth killer, also is very destructive to the body. Over the long term it can cause unnecessary weight gain, leading to diabetes and/or cancer and so many other ills. Sugar generates and feeds gram positive bacteria in the mouth, the bacteria responsible for tooth decay and gum disease. Gram positive bacteria are also responsible for many other diseases of the upper body including acne, tuberculosis, Streptococcus pneumonia, Francisella tularensis, and leprosy. Gram positive bacteria is good in other parts of the body, just not in the mouth.

The healing of teeth is simply having more

of the right bacteria present in your mouth versus the bad bacteria. It's knowing what methods to use that will keep your teeth for as long as you want. A high and properly balanced diet in the right minerals prevents any type of tooth decay that may occur. You only need to know what foods to take, when to take them and how much to take. A high carbohydrate diet has been shown to lead to tooth decay, but the worst offender is processed white sugar and sugary drinks full of calcium draining substances. Researchers have speculated that the mineral content of unrefined carbohydrates prevents bacterial acids from leaching minerals out of the teeth. This is why foods that are unrefined are so much more healthier.

Sometimes you will feel a sore throat coming on if you eat too much sugar, as sugar seems to most affect the upper region of the body. Gram positive bacteria is good in other parts of the body, just not when there is too much of it. There must exist a balance between both the gram positive and gram negative bacteria in order for the body to experience true health.

Dealing with Addictions to Sugar

Over the years, I have found eating chocolate during the winter season to be of benefit. When the weather starts to get warmer, I have found that the chocolate will contribute more than usual to migraines, as well as adverse health effects. This is just my experience and may not be the same to everyone.

I have also noticed over the years that foods that contain sugar create their own self sustaining cycle of psychological addiction to the sugar. This occurs when a person thinks of a sugary food and starts to experience a mouth watering effect in order to satisfy these cravings for sugar.

Why You Crave Sugar

Sugar has actual physical cravings, much

like nicotine. When you think of an item that contains sugar, your mouth waters, which changes the PH of your saliva, as well as many other biochemical changes which take place. This sugar craving is than satisfied by eating foods high in sugar.

This mouth watering method is the same effect used by pizza and pasta restaurants to entice customers. Tomatoes, used in pizza and pasta create a craving via the mouth watering effect. This is than satisfied by eating the pizza dough or pasta, which is high in white flour. Significant long term use of white flour in the diet has long term negative consequences. It also draws out valuable minerals from the body, much like foods high in phytic acids, when eaten and overeating also makes the body acidic.

Methods that Help Eliminate Sugar Cravings

Sugar cravings are 2 fold. They are both Psychological and Physical. Many cravings can be eliminated by changing diet, even for just 48 hours. One technique that works to offset sugar cravings is to take a blank piece of paper and draw a line down the center. Next label one column: benefits of sugar, label the other column, negatives of sugar. Now after writing down the positives and negatives of sugar you will have more will power to overcome the negative effects of sugar intake.

Sometimes this exercise will have more favorable responses than negative ones, however most of the time the responses will be negative, which will reinforce your will power to overcome the urges to eat lots of sugary foods.

Another method that I have found that works is to eat a combination of parsley and yogurt for a couple days in a row and drink lots of spring water. This makes the body more alkaline, which in turn stops the acidic cycle of cravings for sugar and white flour.

Chapter 6

The Importance of Vitamins A, D and K

Scientific Researcher Dr. Weston Price documented the dramatic protective effect of cod liver oil (Vitamins A and D) and butter made from grass fed cows (high in both Vitamins A and K2) against tooth decay. He used a combination of high-vitamin cod liver oil and high-vitamin butter oil to heal cavities, reduce oral gram positive bacteria counts, and cure numerous other afflictions in his patients. Price used extracts from cow butter from cows who ate a diet of green grass in combination with high-vitamin cod liver oil to prevent and reverse dental cavities in many of his patients.

Butter from cows that grazed on grass or open pastures contains numerous beneficial microbes that keep the teeth and gums healthy.

Cod Liver Oil, Raw Organic Butter, Canola Oil and Sunflower Oil are fatty acid oils with long chains. Butter has large amounts of butyric acid, and is a potent antimicrobial and antifungal substance. Butter also contains conjugated linoleic acid (CLA) which gives excellent protection against cancer. Butyric acid is also just starting to be discovered as a powerful anti-aging substance.

Alkaline Proteins, due to their bioavailable calcium content, help keep the teeth healthy. The best one is chlorophyll. (Chlorella, Spinach and Wheatgrass are high in chlorophyll). Research studies show chlorophyll tightens gums, ceases bleeding of gums and forms growth of new gum tissue.

The Miracle of Vitamin K

The proteins in Vitamin K coordinate the movement or organization of calcium. In other situations, the calcium acts as a natural glue, holding the protein in a certain shape. Proteins are only fully functional once they have encountered vitamin K. Vitamin K also works with vitamin D to prevent bone loss and build new teeth and bone. If you are taking antibiotics, be aware that they can destroy vitamin K-producing bacteria in the gut. This effect can be even more powerful if using the cephalosporin class of antibiotics such as cefoperazone (Cefobid®).

K2 is best absorbed into the body with Cod Liver Oil and Organic Butter. It can also be taken with Coconut Oil & Palm Oil. The close cousin to K2, Vitamin K, also can be used for dental health. It works with vitamin D to prevent bone loss and build new bone. Chlorophyll is rich in vitamin K and oxygenates human cells by helping to build red blood cells.

The Best Sources of Vitamin K2

Vitamin K2 is found in the highest levels in Natto. Natto is a type of fermented soybean often served on rice. When you eat it, it 'stretches' like spaghetti, so you have to wrap it around your fork. The best forms of K2 are found almost exclusively in fermented foods.

Vitamin K Foods:

Organic Raw Parsley, Amarath Leaves, Fresh Basil, Sage, Pumpkin Seeds.
A note on Parsley. Some foods that are organic taste so much better and have more nutrients than the non-organic kinds. Parsley is an excellent example. You can readily taste the difference between organic and non-organic parsley.

Cod liver oil, which is high in Vitamins A and D and Parsley or Natto (available in Korean or Japanese Supermarkets) which is high in Vitamin K2 help the body absorb calcium from yogurt.

Cholecalciferol also called vitamin D3 is highest in Raw Mackeral, Raw carp fish and Salted Mackerel.

Vitamin K synergies with Vitamin A and D and Vitamin K2 synergizes with Vitamin D3. Vitamin K2 is found in Butter from grass fed cows.

Lansinoh is an edible form of lanolin or vitamin D3 – you must use an emulsified version or it can make you sick. The best brand is Solgar Vitamin D3 by Biotics research.

Food Sources of K2 from highest to lowest: Parsley Herb (Parsley is super high in Vitamin K, which the body makes into K2), Natto, Goose Liver Paste, Hard Cheeses, Soft Cheeses.

Additional sources of K2 include: Oregano, Cloves, Brussels sprouts, Swiss Chard (raw), Organic Alfalfa, Watercress, Kale, Spinach, Beets, Collards and Chlorophyll.

K2 Synergists include: Cod Liver Oil (fermented Cod Liver Oil works best) & Butter Oil (100% grass-fed, unsalted cultured butter is the best), Vitamins A and D.

The Complete Guide to Natural Toothache Remedies and Re-mineralization

Dairy products rich in this vitamin include egg whites, curd cheeses, butter and whole and low-fat milk.

Spices high in Vitamin K:
Chili Powder (high in Vitamin K and A), Paprika (high in Vitamin K and A), Curry, Cayenne Pepper and Cumin Seed.

If you were to create the ultimate dietary program to immediately heal any cavities, you would want a diet that maximizes the absorption of minerals while providing abundant fat-soluble vitamins. Dr. Price demonstrated that even eating like this for one to two meals a day helps, as you don't have to be totally strict. Below is a guideline you can follow:

Fully pastured dairy products including eggs. Avoid excessive meat.
Fermented grains only. Avoid excessive amounts of oatmeal, breakfast cereals, crackers, etc. Avoid all breads.

Consume nuts and beans in moderation. Nuts and beans are best eaten if soaked overnight or longer, as this significantly reduces their phytic acid content.

Avoid starchy vegetables such as potatoes and sweet potatoes.

Reduce your fruit intake to one piece per day or less.

Vegetables should be lightly steamed.
Try to get good amounts of sunlight, and avoid excessive amounts of sun during the noon time period in summer.

Get proper amounts of high vitamin cod liver oil, and vitamin D3 supplements. Try to avoid the powdered D3, as the gel absorbs much better into the body.
Butter from grass fed cows.

One of the biggest mistakes to make is to continue your diet of eating industrially processed food. This should immediately be ceased if you have a toothache and are healing it.

Chapter 7

The Cause of Toothaches

How To Locate The Foods In Your Diet That Are Contributing To Ill Health

Like we covered in the cavity healing chapter, where changing what you eat, and removing excess processed foods, flours and sugars from the diet will help re-mineralize teeth, the same goes for minor health problems.

Here is a general outline that I successfully follow to keep perfectly healthy:

To name a recent example, while working on the final draft of this book, I developed a lump in my throat that stayed for several weeks. After researching further, I discovered it was called a "Globus mass", which is basically caused by stress. I know from past experience, that diet is the key to healing. So I than replaced 4 main foods from my diet that I commonly ate with 4 other foods for the next 3 days.

I replaced raisins with cranberries, taco shells with sushi, cottage cheese with Swiss cheese and SOD booster mix with more Gotu Kola. The lump faded in 3 days. Over the course of the following week, I than gradually reintroduced the original foods one at time, until I felt the reaction return. I than discovered that the raisins I had been eating had been treated with a new preservative which my body had started to react to, so I than decided to stop eating raisins for a few months.

I have successfully used forms of this over the years to help restore my body back to perfect health. This is a perfect example of instead of going to a costly, time wasting, germ filled emergency room, with a few common sense measures; it saved me time, money and made me wiser.

Foods and Lifestyles that Contribute to Toothaches

In a scientific research study conducted by Dr. T. W. B. Osborn, he discovered that processed wheat and corn flour de-calcify the teeth. This could be due to the phytic acid content of these grains. Pyhtic acid binds minerals and makes them partially unavailable to diffusion into the teeth. This same binding also occurs in the foods we eat. Phytates are not all bad because they can bind to extra iron or toxic minerals in our body and remove them. This allows them to act as chelators, removing excess metals and promoting detoxification. Phytic acid is one of the few chelating therapies used for uranium removal. [15]

It is always better to consume wheat hulls and all, without the bran or the shorts having been removed by the manufacturing process. It is much healthier for you to bake your potatoes with the skins on and then eat them whole. Avoid throwing away the outer leaves of spinach, mustard or lettuce. This is because it is where the nutrient rich layers are.

Some of you reading this may have heard of the famous well-known Pottenger's cat's experiment, which was conducted over several cat generations. The study showed that the cats fed a deficient diet had offspring that were increasingly unhealthy in all respects. Some dentists have also noticed this same trend in dental cavities of families. In families that have several children born close to each other, the best dental health is usually found in the first-born.

Although further research needs to be done, one scientific study suggested that some cancers developing from excess iron, such as colon cancer, that phytic acids help bind to the iron, to prevent the cancer from using the iron to spread by depriving the cancer cells of the iron and similar minerals needed to reproduce. [16]

In an article published by the Journal of Dental Research titled: "A Comparison of Crude and Refined Sugar and Cereals in

Their Ability to Produce in vitro Decalcification of Teeth", which was published in 1937 by Dr. T. W. B. Osborn et al., the scientists studied the South African Bantu and noted their low prevalence of tooth decay. They observed that their diet was high in <u>UNREFINED</u> carbohydrate foods (<u>such as grains that did not have their outer covering removed</u>). When the Bantu was introduced to modern foods such as white flour and refined sugar the rate of decay in their teeth increased rapidly. [17]

Included in the study by Dr. Osborn titled: "A Comparison of Crude and Refined Sugar and Cereals in their Ability to Produce in Vitro Decalcification of Teeth"[18], Dr. Osborn's team decided to do a test on whether refined carbohydrates cause tooth decay. To measure this, the researchers took sets of recently extracted healthy teeth and incubated them with a mixture of human saliva.

They then inserted the following carbohydrate foods into the saliva:

white wheat flour

whole corn meal

refined corn meal

crude cane juice

refined cane sugar

whole wheat flour

The teeth were left incubating with the foods for 2-8 weeks at human body temperature. They also used another set of teeth placed in a saline solution for the control sample. After the study the researchers concluded that the high natural mineral content from the <u>unrefined carbohydrates</u> acted to help prevent the good bacteria from leaching minerals out of the teeth. So in summary we can conclude that unrefined grains are much better for our teeth than over processed grains.

Chapter 8

Weather and Toothaches

Solar Weather and Toothaches

Over the years after checking solar weather in regards to toothache, I discovered that whenever solar activity is stronger, and my body is stressed that I would get a toothache. It is like the solar weather amplifies the stress in the body, thus contributing to increased chances of getting a toothache.

The energy coming from our sun is broken up into a number of different spectrums. These spectrums of energy come from the number of sunspots currently taking place. The spectrum that is responsible for higher levels of stress on the body is increased levels of X-Ray Background Radiation. If we look at Fig 1 on the following pages, we can see that when the X-ray Background Radiation Level is above 4.0, there are more sunspots present. I personally have found that I will experience tooth pain when the x-ray background radiation levels rise above 4.0, especially after the x-ray background radiation levels have been quiet for some time.

Being the founder of the Institute for Solar Studies on Behavior and Human Health I have discovered a link between solar weather and toothaches. There is also a link between terrestrial weather which I will cover shortly. Over the years I had a toothache, they occurred during periods of stronger solar activity. You can plot the time this higher solar activity occurs by looking under the x-ray background section on NOAA's solar weather page and if the x-ray background level has risen above 4.0 or higher, especially for a number of days, your toothaches may get worse. In the photo on the following page there is an illustration of the X-ray background levels. You can get real time solar activity data by visiting the website address below and going to the bottom of the page and clicking on Q1 through Q4.

The Complete Guide to Natural Toothache
Remedies and Re-mineralization

ftp://ftp.swpc.noaa.gov/pub/indices/old_indices/

Quarterly Daily Solar Data

Date	Radio Flux 10.7cm	SESC Sunspot Number	Sunspot Area 10E-6 Hemis.	New Regions	Stanford Solar Mean Field	GOES15 X-Ray Bkgd Flux	C	X-Ray M	X	Flares S	Optical 1	2	3
2015 04 27	108	42	240	0	-999	B2.7	0	0	0	0	0	0	0
2015 04 28	108	36	240	0	-999	B2.7	1	0	0	0	1	0	0
2015 04 29	104	26	30	0	-999	B2.8	1	1	0	0	0	0	0
2015 04 30	102	27	50	2	-999	B2.8	1	0	0	0	0	0	0
2015 05 01	100	13	70	0	-999	B2.2	1	0	0	1	0	0	0
2015 05 02	106	25	220	0	-999	B2.7	0	0	0	6	0	0	0
2015 05 03	111	67	200	3	-999	B4.5	6	0	0	12	1	1	0
2015 05 04	125	85	370	0	-999	B5.6	8	0	0	11	1	0	0
2015 05 05	128	99	650	1	-999	B8.4	18	4	1	17	1	1	0
2015 05 06	136	110	940	0	-999	B8.6	9	1	0	18	1	1	0

Local Weather and Toothaches

As far as localized weather conditions go (terrestrial weather conditions), a rising Dew Point seems to also increase the risk of toothache and abscess formation. It is during these times I have avoided excess sugar intake and detoxed my body more often during these periods to avoid cavities.

A rising Dew Point increases the amount of dampness in the air. If you Google damp weather + toothache, you will see numerous reports of people who experienced toothaches during this period. I believe that this increase in dampness is contributing to or feeding the bacteria that causes toothaches.

During periods of higher solar activity and increased dew point, I have found that oil pulling and removing all high sugar and industrially processed foods from my diet for the next 2 days works extremely well. I have also discovered that foods high in Qucertin, found in large amounts in apples also work well. The food highest in

Quercetin is Capers.

A Dropping Dew Point Leads to Better Health

The Life Fitness Run Club has researched dew point in relation to endurance and discovered that the higher the dew point, than the longer it takes for your sweat to evaporate from your body, thus keeping you cool. This causes your heart and lungs to work harder. This could be that a rising dew point causes less circulation to areas in the upper part of the body, from which antibodies come from the blood to fight infection and disease. Below are the dew points and how they impact endurance provided courtesy of the Life Fitness Run Club.

Dew Point: 50–54 Runner's Perception: Very comfortable How to Handle: Perfect running conditions

Dew Point: 55–59 Runner's Perception: Comfortable How to handle: Hard efforts likely not affected

Dew Point: 60-64 Runner's perception: Uncomfortable for some people How to handle: Expect race times to be slower than in optimal conditions

Dew Point: 65-69 Runner's perception: Uncomfortable for most people How to handle: Easy training runs might feel OK, but difficult to race or do hard efforts

Dew Point: 70-74 Runner's perception: Very humid and uncomfortable How to handle: Expect race paces to suffer greatly

Dew Point: 75 or greater Runner's perception: Extremely oppressive

A dropping dew point I believe increases circulation in the upper part of the body, especially the brain and jaw areas. This is why toothaches are not as common when the dew point is dropping.

So in summary as the dew point rises, it becomes not only more uncomfortable to perform exercises, but the body is more susceptible to tooth infections.

You may find the last few days of Dew Point Activity in your area courtesy of Weather.gov

To locate dew point levels for Portland, OR visit the address below:

http://w1.weather.gov/data/obhistory/KPDX.html

To locate dew point levels for Los Angeles, CA, visit the address below:

http://w1.weather.gov/obhistory/KLAX.html

You can also get a graphical line of dew point activity in your area by entering the following words below into an Internet search engine:

Dew Point + Portland, OR

Besides a rising dew point, another instance where people can experience sudden toothaches from is the condition known as Barodontalgia, also commonly known as "flyers toothache". This results from the sudden pressures experienced during airline flight. In a scientific study titled: "Barodontalgia among flyers: a review of seven cases", advises regular flyers to follow good oral health in order to avoid experiencing Barodontalgia. [19]

Chapter 9

My Personal Experiences of 8 Years of Natural Healing of Toothaches

On November 29th, 2012, while eating, I cracked a tooth, due to a bad filling I had a few years ago. This was at the start of the winter season when warm foods can cause teeth to heat and expand more often than in warmer weather. Instead of going to the dentist and spending large sums of money and go through pain, I decided to apply my knowledge of cavity repair for my broken tooth. A little over 1/3rd of my tooth remains, so repair is possible. At this time I started Oil Pulling with Expeller Pressed Sunflower oil morning, noon and night. I also ate 3 handfuls of raw Parsley throughout the day, because I had no access to Natto,

The next foods high in Natto are Parsley and Sage. I avoided foods containing any sugar for the next 4 days. I also made my body alkaline by taking spring water each morning. After doing this, I also lost my sugar cravings after 3 days.

Within 12 hrs all pain and swelling had subsided and a minor ear infection which had been festering in my right ear, probably due to the tooth infection completely vanished. For dinner for 3 nights in a row I had Plain Organic Yogurt, which is high in Calcium with honey to sweeten it.

Throughout the next 3 days, I always ate 6 handfuls of raw parsley throughout the day. For lunch I had raw sunflower seeds, which remove toxins and are high in Vitamin K and raisins. Twice a day I would take 1 teaspoon of Cod Liver Oil, especially after eating the yogurt. And before bed Spirulina (high in Vitamin A) and raw Sesame seeds (high in calcium).

By the 4th day I could finally grind or pull my teeth together without any more pressure pain and started to return to chewing food on the right side of my mouth.

By day 10, I ate Natto, and Yogurt and drank 1 tablespoon of Cod Liver Oil. By this time, my tooth was at 80% efficiency.

After 2 weeks I could chew properly again without no pain at all and my tooth was 100% painless and fully back to normal functioning where it remains today. (Otober 2015).

I believe because I was taking more Vitamin C than usual due to the start of the flu season, and excess vitamin C depletes calcium levels, this could be what caused my tooth to chip. So I now take more Cod Liver Oil, which also prevents the flu, and take organic foods high in Vitamin C, as well as watch how many Vitamin C tablets I take during the early winter season.

Chapter 10

How to Properly Perform Oil Pulling

In the year 1996, the Indian newspaper Andhra Jyoti held a survey to discover user experiences regarding how effective oil pulling was on their health. From a total of 1041 people who responded, 927 (89%) reported amazing health benefits. The remaining 114 (11%) reported no benefits, possibly due to their bad health, improperly using the oil or other reason.

The survey found oil pulling had the following health benefits.

- Reduced or Eliminated Pains in the body – 758 cases
- Improved the Respiratory system – 191 cases
- Created Healthy Skin – 171 cases
- Improved the Digestive system – 155 cases
- Elimination of Unwanted Unknowns

on the body – 137 cases
- Healed Acing or Sore Joints – 91 cases
- Improved Heart and Circulation – 74 cases
- Reduced Blood Sugar Levels – 56 cases
- Restored Hormones to Healthy Levels – *21 cases*
- *Miscellaneous – 72 cases*

The Miracle of the Sunflower and how it Restores Hormone Levels Naturally

In the relatively new science of Seed Cycling, there is anecdotal evidence stating that eating Sunflower Seeds around a new moon restores hormones to healthy levels. When the full moon occurred, healthy hormones occurred when a person ate pumpkin or flax seeds. Although this science is still early, there is scientific conformation on the effects of oils on the body.

One study done in Australia titled: "A diet rich in high-oleic-acid sunflower oil favorably alters low-density lipoprotein cholesterol, triglycerides, and factor VII coagulant activity", concluded that foods rich in high-oleic-acid sunflower oil was effective in the prevention of heart disease, reduced high cholesterol and reduced blood clots (Factor VII). [20]

In another study titled: "Improvement in HDL cholesterol in postmenopausal women supplemented with pumpkin seed oil: pilot study", [21] researchers found that pumpkin seed oil reduced HDL cholesterol levels in postmenopausal women.

Oil Pulling pulls out toxins from the body, as well as all unwanted matter and toxins from between the teeth. It also feeds the teeth with vital nutrients that create an abundance of good bacteria (the gram negative bacteria) in the mouth. USE COLD PRESSED SUNFLOWER OIL wherever possible, just like un-processed food, cold pressed is more nutrient rich than refined oil. Research has shown that Sunflower or Sesame oils are best. Borage Oil is another beneficial oil for oil pulling.

Oil pulling works best when you make your body more alkaline first, such as can be done by taking Baking Soda or Spring Water before oil pulling. (Aluminum free baking soda is available from Health Food Stores. Bob's Red Mill is one brand).

Here is more detailed information on Oil Pulling from Dr. Karach, the father of Oil Pulling:

"Our research shows that any oil besides SUNFLOWER or SESAME is not effective. On an empty stomach before breakfast, take one tablespoon in the mouth. Move it slowly throughout the mouth in a rinsing and swishing motion. Suck and pull through your teeth for ten to twenty minutes. After a period of time, the oil gets thinner and white. If the oil remains yellow, it has not been pulled through enough. After it starts to turn white, spit it out and do a general rinse with water. One drop of this swished liquid magnified 600 times under a microscope shows toxins and microbes that cause cavities. One of the most beneficial side effects of this is the fastening of loose teeth, and it eliminates bleeding gums and whitens the teeth".

Fast Fact: When you add a very small pinch of Benodite clay *(or French green clay)* to sunflower oil when oil pulling, it greatly synergizes the sunflower oil, enhancing the detoxification and cleansing process. Be sure it is only a very tiny amount of powdered clay as more causes less effectiveness.

Oil pulling is performed best when you allow plenty of oxygen to circulate between the teeth. This means oil pulling outdoors, near an open window, or by breathing deeply in and out a few times as you pull the oil between your teeth.

Another material that is effective for oil pulling is Lecithin. Lecithin allows oil and water to mix more freely, thus allowing easy penetration into the cells of the body. Granulated Lecithin is best. Since

Granulated lecithin is a fat emulsifier, it virtually pulls the bad oils out of the system by literally solubilizing it and the fat is then excreted via the stool, as well as free heavy metals too, which are oil soluble because they are hydrophobic. Take at least 1 tablespoon a day.

Chapter 11

Actions You Can Take to Immediately Relieve a Toothache

A toothache is really the first stage of a mild infection which can grow if not properly treated. Treatment involves a 3 stage process:

1: Eliminating the infection by boosting the immune system with vitamin C or similar.

2: Eliminating the pain with clove, prickly ash or similar numbing herbs.

3: Rebuilding dentin and enamel. This involves adding more calcium and minerals into the diet such as plain Greek yogurt, spirulina, kelp and sea vegetables (which are high in minerals) the herb horsetail (which is high in silica).

A simple example is vitamin C with cod liver oil to remove infection, clove for pain relief and horsetail for rebuilding.

First of all, relax and take off the amount of stress in your body. This involves rest.

Drink plenty of clean and pure water.

The 2 most powerful combinations to stop a toothache immediately are Vitamin K2 and Fermented Cod Liver Oil. The two foods highest in Vitamin K2 are Natto and Kale, especially Kale that has been dried. Natto is made from soybeans that have been fermented and Natto is available from Korean and Japanese Supermarkets.

Vitamin K is best absorbed into the body when taken with Vitamins A and D, which are readily available in cod liver oil.

Get adequate amounts of Qucertin into your body such as from capers or apples. Do not use the supplement qucertin, because it does not dissolve easily into the body. Fom my experience I have found that if the supplement is not fresh, that I have a bad allergic reaction to it, but not to the qucertin occurring in the apples or the capers.

Stop eating all processed foods immediately and go on a mini fast. Increase your intake of lots of spring water or other purified water while fasting.

A mini fast might involve no breakfast and eating 2 grapefruit with honey for lunch while drinking lots of water in-between. Taking a vitamin C capsule (absorbic acid) also creates a synergy with the vitamin C in the grapefruit, boosting the beneficial effects of the grapefruit. (Note: Grapefruit amplifies prescription drugs so be careful if you are taking medication).

Take 2 Carnosine capsules. Also be sure to take a Vitamin D3 GEL capsule with the Carnosine, as Vitamin D3, helps rebuild bone. Take this with 2 tablespoons of honey, which is a powerful natural internal antibiotic. You can also make a more powerful carnosine mix called the Overnight RejuveneEssence Formula as shown in this book.

Take up to 4 ounces of honey over the

next hour. Honey is one of the most powerful killers of bad bacteria in the body.

Perform oil pulling using sunflower oil. Before oil pulling add a very, very tiny pinch of benodite clay to the sunflower oil. After oil pulling for 20 minutes, apply a poultice of benodite clay *(or French green clay)* by mixing the powdered dry clay with a little spring water until it becomes a firm paste. Next holding your mouth open, apply as much of this poultice to the gum line closest to the aching tooth as possible. While holding your mouth open, breath in and out through your mouth and allow the poultice to "harden". Keep on for between 20 to 40 minutes. Rinse mouth thoroughly with warm water, oil pull again and repeat until the pain is gone.

Use mental visualization to see your tooth healing. Just mentally visualize your tooth being surrounded by a golden healing light, nurturing and healing the tooth or a similar image that invites healing.

Recommended Dinner:

You want to have foods that rebuild your gums during this time. The very best combination is sardines mixed with cottage cheese. You will find that after you add the sardines to the cottage cheese that after a few minutes the sardines will "dissolve" into the cottage cheese showing that a beneficial chemical reaction is taking place. The CQ10 in the sardines helps rebuild the gums and the cottage cheese which is high in calcium helps rebuild the gums. Also increasing your intake of calcium with Greek plain yogurt is another way to quickly replenish calcium levels in the body. Plain Greek Organic Yogurt can contain up to 80% calcium. Just sweeten with honey or Steveia.

If available, have Natto 2 times per day. Do this for 4 days in a row and the toothache will have completely disappeared.

I used to use this method when I had dental problems, but now I have adequate amounts of Carnosine which prevents any tooth problems and helps with tooth remineralization.

In Case of Severe Tooth Pain

This method I have used without fail for years.

This method is similar to the previously mentioned method. First make a paste using powered Benodite Clay *(or French green clay)* and Spring Water. Next apply this "putty" mixture over the sore teeth and gum for 20 minutes, than thoroughly rinse mouth with WARM water and repeat at 20 minute intervals if pain still persists. I have also found that adding a few drops of Clove Tincture into the clay also works very well. Clove is an old time tested remedy for toothache. If you don't have a clove tincture you could use clove oil. I have also had good results adding the antibacterial paste Neospoin (*can be found in any good drug store*) to the clay paste works well. This is because

Neosporin fights infection. After removing the clay "putty", oil pull with sunflower oil for best results.

Next we want to re-strengthen the teeth and this can be done by eating Plain Organic Yogurt with Honey to sweeten, and then by eating plenty of Kale or Parsley. These foods are super high in vitamin K and they also pull out metallic toxins from the body.

If you want to go further, than eat pumpkin seeds throughout the day to help flush out parasitic bacteria and drink a combination of apple cider vinegar (diluted in spring water) with garlic and honey throughout the day also helps.

To make drinkable apple cider vinegar, Mix 1/2 gallon of spring water with 3 capfuls of apple cider vinegar, add 3 teaspoons of garlic powder and 4 teaspoons of honey. You can vary the dosages, but this gives you a general idea of how to put the formula together.

The Complete Guide to Natural Toothache Remedies and Re-mineralization

Another good combination is:

Organic yogurt, Cod liver oil, Raw Parsley, Sage Powder, Yogurt, Pumpkin seeds, Spirulina, Sesame seeds and Parsley. Take at least a full bunch of parsley for 3 days in a row with yogurt and cod liver oil for best results.

The best way to get the best results is to take lots of vitamin d and vitamin k with organic calcium from plain Greek yogurt. Cod liver Oil is high in Vitamin A. Spirulina is high in Vitamin A.

The above methods have always relieved any toothache or severe gum infection within 24 hours or less without fail.

You can find literally thousands of testimonials and user experiences from people who have used this combination by doing an Internet Search for "apple cider vinegar and garlic toothache", showing how effective garlic is as a natural antibiotic.

Why Cinnamon is More Effective than Clove in Reducing or Eliminating Toothache. The Scientific Evidence

In a science research study titled: "Comparative Study Of Cinnamon Oil And Clove Oil On Some Oral Microbiota." [29] researchers compared the effectiveness of cinnamon oil to clove oil and found that cinnamon oil worked better than the clove oil at reducing negative oral microbiota. Cinnamon has also been found to be effective in reducing or eliminating bad breath and lowering high blood sugar. In the case of using herbal tinctures, they absorb better into the body when placed directly under the tongue for 20 to 45 seconds.

Herbs and Compresses for Immediate Pain Relief

Prickly Ash, Kava or Spilanthes. For best results drop an alcohol extract directly on the tooth.

Make a warm compress of warm Ginger and apply to the cheek area nearest the toothache.

Use the below formula and massage into receding gums, increase circulation, tighten tissues and decrease bad microbes:

2 parts Yerba mansa
1/2 part myrrh
2 parts echinacea
2 parts prickly ash bark

You can also use the above as a mouth rinse by running it through a water pik which is a oral irrigation device that puts out a stream of water to gently massage in-between the teeth and gums.

Prickly Ash.

This herb has a very similar effect to the substance novocaine, which is used to temporarily to numb tissues. The bark is ground up, made into a poultice and applied to toothaches. Prickly Ash makes a great way to instantly remove a toothache while you can apply more intensive tooth healing methods in the meantime, such as making your body alkaline and boosting your immune system.

Using Ormus to help Relieve a Toothache

Before I started taking Carnosine, I used other techniques to help get rid of toothaches. For those of you who are not familiar with Ormus, it is a special mixture made up of certain elements that react favorably with good bacteria in our body. It can be used both internally and externally. I have used it over the years for many things, and it is especially good for teeth. An Internet search term Ormus + Teeth yields many people who have found using Ormus with toothpaste to be a great way to keep teeth and gums healthy.

Chapter 12

Using Hydrogen Peroxide for Dental Hygiene and Health

The first use of hydrogen peroxide in dentistry was first recorded in the year 1913. It was used to decrease plaque formation and also used to control "pyorrhea" or gum disease.

Hydrogen Peroxide works wonders for the teeth and gums because it is a natural germ killer. Hydrogen peroxide is also a convenient source of oxygenated water. You can also use it to disinfect your toothbrush before or after brushing. Hydrogen peroxide works best when diluted with water. Use the following amounts of hydrogen peroxide diluted with water for best results:

For an abscessed gum, soak a cotton ball with diluted hydrogen peroxide (add 1% to 3% of hydrogen peroxide to water). You may also want to add a drop of clove to the cotton ball.

As a mouth wash and gargle (disinfectant) (add 1% to 3% of hydrogen peroxide to water).

As a tooth paste, mixed with baking soda (add 1% to 3% of hydrogen peroxide to water).

Herbs for Mouth Rinses

The herbs Goldenseal, Oregon Grape and Barberry can not only freshen breath and keep bad bacteria at bay, they can also be used as a sore/strep throat gargle.

How to Make Your Own Natural Breath Freshener

Bad breath comes from bacteria that gather and get stuck on the tongue and also from food particles that get stuck between the teeth. It can also come from poor eating habits. Here is an excellent remedy to help get rid of the bad bacteria and bad breath.

Fill 1/2 cup water and add 4 drops of anise essential oil, 4 drops fennel essential oil, 4 drops cinnamon essential oil and 4 drops of peppermint essential oil or tea tree oil than rinse out the mouth.

Chapter 13

Proven Techniques and Methods that Heal Dental Abscesses

If your toothache persists long enough and you have not taken adequate steps to boost your immune system, such as taking extra vitamin C or Garlic, an abscess will start to form. This can than create an infection that can spread to other parts of your body. The infection than begins to reduce blood circulation reducing your flow of blood, which leads to clogged arteries and eventually kills you.

How Gum Disease Increases Your Chances of a Stroke

Bacterial infections cause changes in the body's chemistry, creating a predisposition to thrombosis (clotting). If the infection is chronic it can cause atherosclerosis, which is how the immune system handles infection. Over time this gradually contributes to an increase of bad bacteria in the blood supply. This could cause the body to succumb to a toxic bacterial infection. In a 1997 scientific study titled: "Inflammation, aspirin, and the risk of cardiovascular disease in apparently healthy men", published by the National Institute of Health, researchers found that inflammation increased the chances of stroke in healthy men.

In another study titled: "Relationship between periodontal disease, tooth loss, and carotid artery plaque: the Oral Infections and Vascular Disease Epidemiology Study (INVEST)" published in 2003, researchers studied 711 people with a mean age of 66 years. The study found that tooth loss can increase the rate of subclinical atherosclerosis in the body.

How to use Niacin (vitamin B3) to Heal an Abscess

In a 2012 study published by researchers from Cedars-Sinai Medical Center in California which was published in the Journal of Clinical Investigation, researchers studied human blood and living mice and found that that mice who were deficient in vitamin B3 suffered more frequent severe infections. If the mice were given high doses of vitamin B3 before they were exposed to an infectious bacteria, the infection developed, however it cleared much more quickly. Another interesting discovery is when the mice were given vitamin B3 after their infections, their infection cleared much more quickly. This only occurred however, in mice that had adequate levels of vitamin B3 before their clinically induced infection.

The best dose to start with is to take between 50mg and 100mg Vitamin B3 every 1 to 2 hours or so. This will help remove congested blood in the area of an infection out of the area, re-promoting healthy blood flow.

Some people have had success taking Niacin before going into a sauna. This is because saunas help remove toxins and increase circulation, due to the high heat causing the heart to work harder.

During a Longevity Conference hosted by nutrition expert David Wolfe, Dr. Yu stated at the conference that the best method is to begin with low amounts of niacin such as 50 milligrams if your body okays the tolerance, and then to build up to 500 milligrams. Studies have proven that people who had Gulf War Syndrome tolerated up to 5000 mgs.

Saunas increase the body temperature, which causes the immune system to strengthen itself and flush out toxins via a stronger heart rhythm. Many people claim a niacin and sauna detoxification really has a positive effect. Some people have added Bentonite clay, parsley and Zeolite before taking the sauna. Vitamin B3 (Niacin) is a water soluble vitamin, so high doses of niacin are relatively safe. High doses have been used in orthomolecular medicine and psychiatry since the late 1950s for depression and anxiety.

Propolis.
Propolis is also known as bee glue and is a resinous substance that bees collect from sap flows, tree buds, and similar botanical sources. It is a powerful natural healing substance made by bees that has powerful benefits on the upper part of the body. Because honey is one of nature's most powerful internal natural antibiotics, it would only make sense that Propolis would fight bad bacteria, fungi and infection. Use Propolis to help heal an infection caused by a toothache if your tooth has gotten really bad. You can also use it for sore throats. To use for a toothache, apply between one and two drops directly on the tooth. Do this twice daily and the infection should be gone within three days or less.

In a scientific research study titled: "Propolis: A New Alternative for Root Canal Disinfection" [32] researchers discovered that when they compared propolis with calcium hydroxide (*aka Edible Lime, Hydrated Lime, CaH2O2*), that it was more powerful than calcium at eliminating certain germs. So this would make an excellent remedy for a tooth that may require a "root canal".

For excessive inflammation of the gums, use a hot compress or poultice of equal parts of milky oats, chamomile and bergamot flowers.

Using a Ginger and Mustard Footbath for Pain Relief

A hot foot bath with Ginger or Mustard powder draws pain away from the jaw. Soak your feet in the solution for 3 minutes and then plunge your feet in cold water for about a minute. Rotate every 15 minutes for best results. If you continue for longer than 20 minutes, add some salt to the foot bath to remove any bad bacteria that may build up.

How to use Golden Seal and Myrrh

The herbs Golden seal and myrrh are commonly used as a natural disinfectant. They can also be placed into capsules or made into a tincture to help heal an infection.

Pine Tree Resin

When the resin from a pine tree is made into a poultice and placed next to an abscess it will help to draw out infection.

Potassium chloride

Potassium chloride (kali mur) is cell salt number 4 in Europe. In the US, Potassium chloride (kali mur) is cell salt number 5. Use for severe tooth infections. It is effective against pus pockets in the tooth roots and infections in the jaw.

Cepacol

Many people have had success with Cepacol. You can purchase Cepacol as a mouth rinse. Just gargle with Cepacol in the mouth for 5 minutes at regular times throughout the day until the abscess has relieved itself.

Be sure to drink plenty of water throughout the day to flush your body free of the toxins and bad bacteria generated by the abscess.

Petasites or Butterbur (Petasites hybridus / officinalis)

Invented by Swiss naturopath Dr. H.C. Alfred Vogel Petaforce, these capsules have extraordinary strong analgesic properties. In one case Pastor Soeken took six Petaforce capsules before having his tooth pulled out and did not need anesthesia.

On the website www.erapy.co.uk/information/conditions_p

ainrelief.html one writer stated that Petaforce is one of the fastest-acting pain killers due to its fast acting analgesic action which occurs within just twenty to thirty minutes. Petasites will strengthen the heart and is endorsed by The American Academy of Neurology and the American Headache Society for use in natural prevention of migraines.

Asafoetida

This is another heart strengthening herb which is commonly used in India. To use, boil half a teaspoon of asafoetida in a cup of water. After the water cools to room temperature, make into a poultice and place it on the inflamed tooth. Hold the poultice to the tooth as long as you feel comfortable, than thoroughly rinse your mouth out and do oil pulling. You can use the remaining asafetida water as a mouth rinse by gargling with it 2 to 3 times daily.

Swedish bitters (herbal remedy)

This is a common cure all for numerous physical ailments. To use, add 1 tablespoon of Swedish Bitters to water and hold in the mouth for a while. You may also want to moisten the gum first with the essential oil of Wintergreen, some drops of a herbal tincture of Cajuput or by rinsing the mouth with ginger water first. These will moisten the gums and allow the Swedish Bitters to more thoroughly penetrate into the gum.

You can also make your own Swedish Bitters tincture, which you can find in my book: The Official Guidebook of How to Make Tinctures and Alchemy Spagyric Formulas (*available on Amazon.com*)

As previously covered in this book, for an abscessed gum you can use diluted hydrogen peroxide. Just soak a cotton ball with diluted hydrogen peroxide (add 1% to 3% of hydrogen peroxide to water). You may also want to add a drop of clove to the cotton ball.

The Chinese herb Baizhi (common name Angelica) can be used for severe tooth abscesses. It works also to relieve headache. It induces perspiration, expels wind and relieves pain.

Goldenseal tincture

Apply a few drops of Goldenseal tincture to your tooth to help alleviate toothache.

Edible Bentonite Clay and Mineral Rich French Green Clay

Bentonite Clay and French Green Clay both have high natural electrical charges. Due to this negative charge, the clay helps to draw out toxins and infection from the gums. Most toxins in the body hold a positive charge. If you introduce Bentonite Clay (which is edible) into the body, which is negatively charged, the positively charged toxins adhere to the clay, drawing out the toxins. This works much like a magnet, where the negative pole attracts the positive pole. The darker the Green in the Clay, the more mineral rich it is. French Green Clay happens to be of a dark green, compared to the powdery white clay of Bentonite.

Bentonite Clay and French Green Clay are available in a powder from most natural food stores. I usually do 1 sunflower oil pulling with a touch of clay and 2 oil pullings without. Too much clay mixed with sunflower oil seem to hinder the beneficial effects.

Frankincense. (Boswellia Carterii).
A powerful antibacterial. It also increases circulation, making it great for removing the final stages of a dental abscess.

Tea Bags
You can also place a tea bag on the tooth or soak the tea bag for 5 minutes in any of the above mentioned herbal remedies and apply to the tooth.

How To Make A Poultice Using Tea Bags
Tea bags make a great poultice, because the bags easily soak up herbs. To make a poultice, place a tea bag in hot water, then add herbs, gently stir and soak for 3 to 5 minutes. Next remove the tea bag and place on gum closest to the aching tooth.

Rapid Toxin Removal

Toxins, especially those that have built up in your body from various metals contained in the air and food must be flushed as quickly and as thoroughly from your body as soon as possible during your "healing process". Besides Niacin, which we covered earlier, the two best substances are Zeolite, including the Zeolite mix which we show how you can make at the end of this book, and raw organic parsley. With Zeolite you just mix the powder with warm water until it is fully dissolved and drink it with plenty of water. Using parsley, you can eat it directly with yogurt, or you can boil up some hot water and soak the parsley directly in the hot water for a few minutes and then drink it directly. This parsley water is also very good for the heart.

A Formula For Relief of Inflamed Gums

Pour 1 cup of boiling water over 1 tablespoon of the herb sage and then cover and steep for 25 minutes and then strain. Next add 2 tsp of sea salt. To use, rinse mouth with this solution after brushing teeth.

Chapter 14

Methods to Fight Infection and Boost the Immune System while Alleviating Toothache

Chamomile is an amazing herb, because unlike Echinacea, which can only be used in small amounts, Chamomile can be used in higher dosages to help fight infection and create a sedative like effect on the body. It also has uses both internally and externally. To prepare, steep between 1/2 and 1 cup of Chamomile flowers in boiling hot water, wait 10 minutes until it has cooled down than slowly drink. Drink 3 cups of Chamomile tea a day to fight infection and help speed your healing.

Chamomile can also be used externally when combined with Goldenseal and Clove. To use, combine the following ingredients together until a thick paste forms:

1 drop of clove essential oil
2 drops of chamomile essential oil
1/2 tsp goldenseal powder

Next dab the paste onto the tooth to relieve pain instantly. You may have to keep your mouth open a couple of minutes to evaporate saliva so that the paste adheres more firmly to the tooth, or you may want to mix it with some benodite *(or French green clay)* clay to create a putty like substance.

White Oak Bark

This herb is the main secret contained in Dr. Christopher's herbal tooth and gum powder. White Oak Bark helps set/tighten teeth that are loose. Some people have used it by applying oak bark powder between the gums and cheeks before bed to tighten the teeth. Use for firm gums and strong teeth.

Boosting Your Immune System

When your body is fighting an infection, your immune system is working extra hard. Be sure to get rest, drink plenty of water and to take adequate amounts of Zinc and Vitamin C. If you are using the herbs Echinacea or Spilanthes, these herbs automatically boost your immune system, while at the same time relieve your toothache so they make good herbs if your immune system is weak. If you feel extreme inflammation coming on, take willow bark tea, as this will naturally help fight inflammation.

Chapter 15

Foods for Healthy Teeth

Let's recap on the methods covered so far. The most common foods for healthy teeth are:

Organic yogurt

Cod liver oil

Organic Raw Parsley

Sage Powder

Pumpkin seeds

Spirulina

Sesame seeds

Cod liver Oil. (is high in Vitamin A)

Spirulina. (is high in Vitamin A and minerals)

Chapter 16

Cell Salts Known to Relieve Toothache

Cell salts were invented by the German physician Dr. Wilhelm Heinrich Schubler (1821–1898). They are based on inorganic mineral salts. According to Schubler's research, the body sometimes undergoes an imbalance or deficiency of the 12 salts in the body, which occur at the cellular level. This imbalance can lead to sickness. Cell Salts work best taken in hot water between 3 and 4 p.m. in the afternoon, when the body is naturally warmer, allowing for complete absorption of the cell salts. Cell Salt tablets can be purchased on Amazon or any other reputable merchant.

Instructions for making a cell salt solution: Place between 3 and 10 tablets in a 16 to 24 ounce bottle. Next fill with water and gently swirl the tablets to dissolve them thoroughly. The solution will keep long enough that you can sip the water throughout the day.

Potassium Chloride (Kali Mur) –
Potassium chloride (kali mur) is cell salt number 4 in Europe. In the US, Potassium chloride (kali mur) is cell salt number 5. Use for severe tooth infections. It is effective against pus pockets in the tooth roots and infections in the jaw. It has no side effects when responsibly used.

To use; place ten tablets in a cup of hot water, wait a few minutes until dissolved. Once dissolved, sip slowly and repeat several times a day. If you see no result it is because you did not take enough. Don't worry about overdosing, I personally have never heard of a cell salt overdose. With regular intake and proper nutrition, the pus pocket will heal.

Calcium fluoride (calc fluor)
Calcium fluoride Tissue salt number 1, Calcium fluoride (calc fluor). This cell salt will help with defective tooth enamel. Some people have claimed it caused

cavity reversal. It is used by placing between three and four tablets directly on the toothache (*preferably on the root of the tooth*) several times throughout the day and before bed.

Magnesia Phosphoria. Works well for toothaches, sensitive teeth or teething pains.

Additional Cell Salts for alleviating Toothache

Calc Fluor 6X – Supports teeth enamel and eliminates pain upon eating

Calc phos 6X – Helps increase calcium absorption, and eliminates particularly serious toothaches accompanying a swollen cheek

Ferr phos 6X – Use for inflammation or toothache caused after eating food

Mag phos 6X – For sharp shooting pains or cold environments that cause toothache

Chapter 17

Use the Power of Your Mind to Heal a Toothache

Tooth nerves are unique compared to other parts of the body. This is because these nerves are closest to the pain centers of our brain compared to the nerves in other part of our body. Some people have expressed that their toothaches simply "vanished" when they made an appointment to see their dentist. Other people felt an immediate sense of calm after having talked to someone about their toothache. Could there be some type of emotional connection between the nerves in our teeth and the chemicals that govern our emotions? Could emotional relief be creating some sort of natural painkiller? Other people have shared experiences where they used sheer willpower and concentration to alleviate the pain of their toothache.

Because my research has proven that Psychosomatic illness (you belief makes you think u are sick) occurs most often when the sun's x-ray background radiation levels are dropping below 4.0, this would be the best time to use mind visualization to relieve toothache.

The best method that I have found when a toothache becomes unbearable is to use the benodite clay technique mentioned earlier in this book and to visualize oneself already being relieved of pain and being at peace. It helps to visualize the tooth surrounded in a glowing healing golden orb of light, mending and soothing the tooth. Because we are working with nerves, it also helps to simply and firmly tell the toothache to leave.

The Connection Between Stress and Toothaches

People most vulnerable to toothache are those with teeth that have had dental work done on them, or may have a cracked tooth or other tooth abnormality. When a toothache forms in these vulnerable regions of the mouth. This occurs because the root-canalled tooth or other previously repaired tooth consists of "*dead*" tissue. Because of the body's automatic healing process, the body will attempt to gradually decompose this dead tissue (*tries to get rid of it*) via bacterial lysis. This process is similar to how your body reacts when a splinter gets lodged under your skin. Your body gradually rejects it, pushing it to the surface. This is because it is a dead foreign object.

How Stress can Bring on a Toothache

From reading of the experiences of others, and from my own experiences I can assure you that stress can indeed bring on a toothache. This must also mean that removing stress from our life temporarily will help heal a toothache, which I have found to be true.

The Complete Guide to Natural Toothache Remedies and Re-mineralization

The pain of experiencing toothache itself is a big stressor and combined with feelings of helplessness will increase the stress even more. If the body is overstressed, symptoms can include bruxism (*the continuous grinding of one's teeth*). The teeth can experience up to 400 g of pressure from the constant grinding motion. The best way to remove stress quickly is to get away from the situation that is causing you undue stress. Take some time off and get some rest and eat nutritious foods and get some fresh air and sunshine. Doing this for just 48 hours along with the various toothache relief formulas found in this book will work wonders.

Chapter 18

Natural Herbs for Gums with Inflammation and Bleeding Gums

The main cause for unhealthy gums is a diet lacking in adequate minerals. Sea minerals, found in abundant levels in spirulina and other sea algae foods, contain minerals tiny enough to be properly and rapidly absorbed by the mouth and body, helping to attack the bad bacteria and strengthen the good bacteria. This is why foods that are high in minerals work wonders at stopping gums that are bleeding.

Himalayan Salt

Himalayan Salt, which is one of the few foods packed densely with minerals helps stop bleeding gums. Himalayan salt is made up of 84 minerals. It also contains the elements such as hydrogen and oxygen. In a repot titled: "Certificate of the

Analysis of the Original Himalayan Crystal Salt Institute of Biophysical Research, Las Vegas, Nevada, USA June 2001 (*You can download the report for free*), the report showed in their spectral analysis that Himalayan salt contained both of the major macro minerals calcium and chloride, and it had abundant sources of trace minerals such as iron and zinc.

To use Himalayan Salt to stop bleeding gums, add one teaspoon of Himalayan salt to 1 cup of warm water, allowing the crystals to fully dissolve. Next gargle with it. This mouthwash can also be used to get rid of bad breath. If your gums are sore, bleeding or you have an oral infection, then rinse with warm water with Himalayan Salt three to four times daily.

Use Vitamin C in Grapefruit to Stop Bleeding Gums

As mentioned earlier, the more bio-available the vitamins or minerals are, the better they are for your health. Grapefruit happens to be very high in bio-available Vitamin C. Researchers from the Friedrich Schiller University in Germany found that people with gum disease had significantly less bleeding when they ate two grapefruits a day for two weeks. The study also showed it reduced inflammation caused by gum disease. The full study was conducted by Dr Gordon Watkins of the Friedrich Schiller University in Germany and is published in the British Dental Journal. The study involved 58 people that had chronic gum disease. [30]

This is why you would not want to depend on vitamin C tablets (ascorbic acid) because the molecules in them are not tiny enough to be properly absorbed by the mouth and body, compared to the vitamin C molecules that are smaller and more totally absorbed by the body when eating Grapefruit.

As we covered earlier, Vitamin D3 drops or D3 gel caps are better for the body because they are absorbed more completely into the body, allowing your body to properly get adequate doses of the Vitamin and use it properly. In a scientific study titled: "Comparative Bioavailability To Humans Of Ascorbic Acid Alone Or In A Citrus Extract" [31] researchers discovered that when a liquid extract of Vitamin C was used, it absorbed more thoroughly into the body than just plain Vitamin C tablets. Most of the Vitamin C tablets you buy in the store are nothing more than ascorbic acid powder dried into a tablet.

Herbs for Healthy Gums

Marshmallow.
Chew the herb or apply directly to the gum and tooth area to help relieve toothache.

Nutmeg.
Add 1 or 2 drops of essential oil of nutmeg to gumline of tooth.

Elecampane.
Mix with essential oil and apply directly to the gums.

Quick Methods that Stop Bleeding Gums

By adding a little bit of DMSO (*a compound that naturally absorbs through the skin into the bloodstream*), it has been shown to heal abscessed teeth. Some people have used it to successfully treat tumors both inside the body or topically. Some people mix it with colloidal silver. A good remedy is 2-3 oz. of hot/warm water and then place 2 tablespoons of 10ppm colloidal silver in the water. Next add 6 drops of DMSO. Keep in your mouth 2-3 minutes then spit out. Use 2 to 3 times a day.

Herbs for Relief of Periodontal Disease

The best herbs for Periodontal Disease include: Goldenseal, Ginkgo, Spilanthes, Echinacea, Oregon Grape or Barberry. Garlic and Vitamin E also help reduce infection.

Chapter 19

The Complete Master Herbal List for Alleviating Toothaches

Cow Parsnip (Heracleum maximum (H lanatum). Make into a polutice and place directly on toothache.

Ground Ivy (Glechoma hederacea, Nepeta hederacea). This herb works on the upper part of the body. It is ground up and used for toothache and headaches.

Houseleek (Sempervivum tectorum). The leaves of this herb are chewed to relieve toothache.

Hops (Humulus lupulus). Due to its mildly sedative and diuretic properties, it is commonly used for toothache.

Horsetail. One of the more popular herbs is Horsetail. This is because Horsetail contains high levels of the mineral Silica. Many people are confused as to how much horsetail delivers the best results. The best results seem to be several grams a day for the best effects. This is because it assists in bone growth, rather than acting as a nutrient.

Comfrey Root. This herb works best when used with bentonite clay *(or French green clay)* as a poultice on the exterior of the teeth.

WinterGreen. Early American settlers used this herb by having their children chew the roots of Wintergreen for 6 weeks at the start of spring. The berries are steeped in brandy and used as a winter tonic. Wintergreen is used in many mouthwashes to kill bad bacteria in the mouth. It also comes in an essential oil. Other uses include as a skin softener and it eases muscular, arthritic and rheumatic pains due to its ability to rapidly penetrate the skin. It is commonly used as a natural flavoring for toothpaste and has multiple uses in the dental ceramics industry.

Borage. Borage has shown potential in treating periodontitis (*gum disease*) and gingivitis. Some people have used a mixture of Borage and Spirulina for healthy gums.

Leadwort (Plumbago europaea). Chewing the root of this plant causes the mouth to produce excess amounts of saliva. Place near gum to treat toothache. The dried root also makes a great natural chewing-gum. Poultices of this plant are also used to heal back pain and sciatica. Its traditional use is for epilepsy and scabies.

Marigold. This plant is also used for sore eyes. To prepare for healing teeth, add 0.5oz of dried flower heads of marigold and boil in water. Next allow to cool and drink or apply to the tooth.

Another Marigold preparation consists of mixing the petals with vinegar and rubbing into the gums for pains of the teeth. Marigold is also planted in gardens to be used as a powerful natural insect repellent. It can also be used for sore or red eyes.

Sesame seeds. Because sesame oil is used for oil pulling, the seeds can be used for swollen gums. To prepare, boil 1 part sesame seeds in 2 parts of water until there is 1 part of water remaining. Next use the liquid used as a gargle. This is reported to be a very powerful remedy. Use with oil pulling for maximum results.

Coriander Seeds. To use, take 0.3oz of coriander seeds and boil down to about 1 quart and use as a mouth rinse.

Watermelon Rind. To use, burn dried watermelon until it becomes an ash. Next place a tiny amount of ash on gum line closet to the aching tooth.

Ginger. The powder of Ginger is applied directly to the tooth in a poultice. Ginger has muscle relaxing properties. It makes a great way to open the pores of the gums before rinsing or treating them with herbs. You can also warm the ginger beforehand by placing a tea bag in warm water, adding some ginger. Once the ginger has dissolved into the tea bag, place next to the aching tooth.

Ground apricot kernels or Apricot Kernel Powder (*which you can buy on Amazon*) has a mild numbing effect, helping to relieve toothache.

Pasque Flower (Pulsatilla vulgaris). Used to treat toothache, this herb also has multipurpose properties. Other uses include: as a sedative for sleep difficulties, cataracts, inflammatory conditions, nervousness, despondency, sadness, unnatural fear, weepiness and depression, headache and insomnia,

Pellitory of the Wall (Parietaria officinalis). This plant loves to grow on walls and locations where there is lots of stone. Because it loves hard locations, this could be why it hardens teeth. This root can be taken as a decoction or chewed to relieve toothache. When diluted with a carrier oil (such as jojoba) it can be massaged into the gum closest to the aching tooth. When mixed with distilled water, Pellitory of the Wall can be used as a mouthwash. The decoction is also used as a gargle to soothe sore throats. Like Leadwort, it will increase the amounts of saliva in the mouth.

Pepper (Piper nigrum). Used to help reduce toothache pain.

Periwinkle (Vinca Major and V minor). The roots of this plant are chewed for toothache.

Red Cedar. The leaf buds are chewed to relieve toothache.

Rhatany (Krameria triandra). Commonly used in herbal toothpastes and powders. It is very good at healing bleeding gums due to its powerful astringent properties. It is commonly mixed with bloodroot and used as a snuff to treat nasal polyps.

Rooibos (Aspalathus linearis). I have used this tea myself personally for many years, and found it greatly strengthens the gums, and it also inhibits bad bacteria in the mouth that cause tooth decay. It is also caffeine-free, meaning you get lots of energy from it without the sugar crash. Roobios tea is one of the few herbs that contains high levels of natural fluoride. The best roobios tea is the unfermented shoot and leaf teas. Do not use the bagged versions of Roobios as they have less nutrients.

Scurvy Grass (Cochlearia officinalis). An effective toothache reliever, an infusion is made of this consisting of 8 parts leaves, 3 parts alcohol and 3 parts water. This is than concentrated to two-thirds of its original volume. Make into a poultice or soak on a cotton ball and apply directly to tooth.

Sumac, Smooth (Rhus glabra). The sap of this plant is placed directly on an aching tooth. Infusions of Sumac are also used for relieving rheumatism and aching muscles.

<u>Handy Hint: To brew loose leaf tea, place herbs in a tea ball, tea filter or strain the hot tea through a very fine strainer into a cup.</u>

Sweet Sumach (Rhus aromatica). The fruit of Sweet Sumach is highly astringent. The fruits are chewed to relieve toothaches, gripe and stomach aches. It can also be made into a gargle to treat mouth and throat complaints.

Szechuan Pepper (Zanthoxylum piperitum (Xanthoxylum piperitum). This plant is related to prickly ash, another toothache relieving plant. Make into a poultice and apply to toothache.

Tarragon (Artemisia dracunculus). This herb is chewed thoroughly to numb a toothache. It can also be taken before ingesting a bitter medicine. Other uses include insomnia, and in warmer climates it is used to treat threadworms in children.

Tea Tree. Can be diluted in vegetable or jojoba oil at 5% for massaging into gums. Also used as a gargle for mouth ulcers, toothaches, and bad gums. Tea tree is also used for Acne, in conjunction with debridement; Pharyngitis; Sinusitis and Tinea pedis, also known as athlete's foot by massaging into the feet and toes daily.

Toad Herb (Franseria tenuifolia (syn Ambrosia tenuifolia). This root is ground up and placed into tooth cavities for relief of toothache. The leaves, either green or dried and ground, is made into a tea and used for stomach distress.

Bhringraj (Trailing Eclipta (Eclipta prostrata (syn E. alba)). The roots of this are ground into a powder and mixed with pepper and then applied to toothache for relief.

Additional Uses: Use as a mouth rinse to keep away toothaches, oral infections and strengthen gums and teeth. Place 4 drops of an extract of Bringraj in the opposite ear a toothache is present. For example, if the pain is in left side of the face then place drops in the right side ear and vice versa.

Vervain (Verbena officinalis). Has effects very similar to aspirin, but biochemically has a much different structure than aspirin. Has many multipurpose uses. Very effective at relieving inflammation, treating headaches, toothaches and wounds.

Yarrow (Achillea millefolium). The fresh leaves of Yarrow are chewed to relieve toothache.

Yellow Poplar (Liriodendron tulipifera (syn Tulipifera liriodendron)). The bark contains high levels of 'tulipiferine', which stimulates the heart and nervous systems. A decoction of the root bark of this plant is applied warm to an infected tooth for immediate relief of pain. An ointment can be made by crushing the buds in grease and treating scalds, burns, and inflammations. Crushed leaves are used in a poultice to treat headaches. Externally the tea can be made into a wash and used as a poultice on wounds and boils. The root bark and seeds can be used to expel worms from the body.

Cumin Seed. A great spice that also greatly helps reduce sugar and junk food cravings by taking 3 to 5 teaspoons of cumin powder in a cup of water. This spice also helps treat tooth decay, and reduces toothache. It is commonly used in tooth powders and mouth rinses.

Coriander Seeds. Take 0.3oz of coriander seeds and place in boiling water until about 1 quart of water remains. Next use as a mouth rinse.

Fennel Seed. Used to make toothpaste.

Areca Nut (Areca catechu) – Ayurveda medicine recommends burning this nut until it becomes charcoal and then mixing with a quarter part of powdered cinnamon to produce a powerful healing tooth powder. Also a decoction made from the root of this nut is good for sore lips. In Traditional Chinese Medicine. Fennel moves chi downwards and eliminates food stagnation and assists digestion. It has mild toxic properties and should be taken in moderation.

Aztec Sweet Herb (Phyla scaberrima). To use for toothaches, the flowers are chewed or can be directly placed upon the gum.

Bai Zhi (Angelica Root). This herb has been used for thousands of years in Chinese herbal medicine. It is a sweat-inducing herb used to counter harmful external influences. It acts on the upper part of the body helping to relieve headaches, aching or sore eyes, nasal congestion and toothache.

Myrrh. Has been valued for thousands of years for its ability to fight infections of the mouth including gum disease, bad breath, toothache and for a healthy throat and sinus.

Spilanthes. (Spilanthes Acmella). This plant is commonly called Toothache plant. It is a natural strong anti inflammatory and antimicrobial.

Frankincense. (Boswellia Carterii). A powerful antibacterial. It also increases circulation, making it great for removing the final stages of a dental abscess. To use, mix Frankincense with Myrrh for gingivitis, inflammation of the gums and loose tooth sockets. Can be used topically for sores.

Chapter 20

Understanding How Teeth Remineralize Themselves

Decay of teeth is caused by acidic saliva. This is because the demineralization of enamel occurs at the pH value below 5.5. This means that if your diet consists of high amounts of white flour, processed foods and the like, your saliva will most likely be acidic, contributing partly to dental decay. The PH of your saliva varies throughout the day, with the early morning and late night hours being most alkaline. If we look at a Stephen Curve PH Chart shown on the next page, we can see the varying PH level of PH in the mouth. The higher the line, the more alkaline.

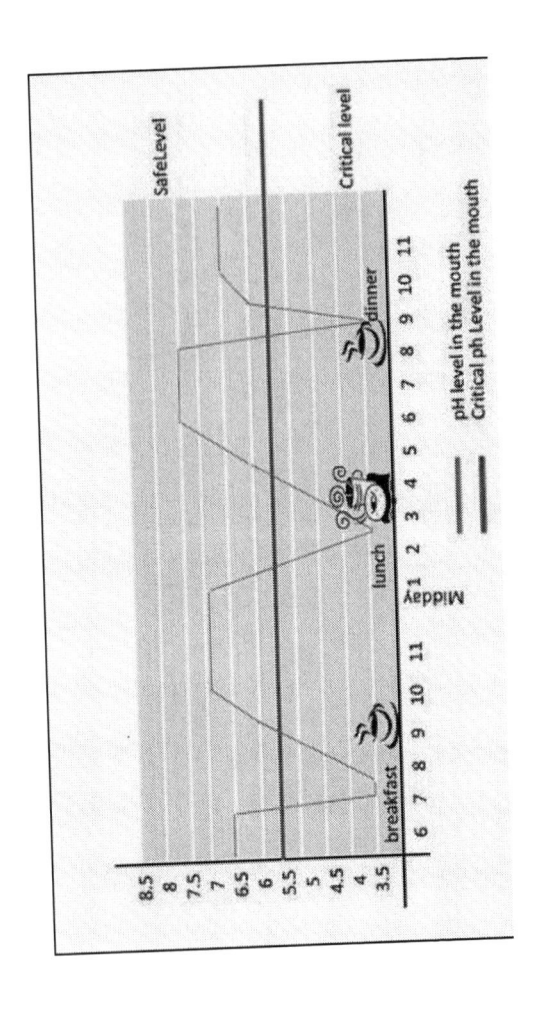

The main bacteria responsible for tooth decay are the cocci shaped gram positive bacteria Streptococcus mutans [36] and lactobacillus bacteria. When the saliva has a PH of between 6.8 and 7.4, which

The Complete Guide to Natural Toothache Remedies and Re-mineralization

occurs when you eat calcium rich foods and alkaline foods, the minerals in the foods such as calcium, phosphate, and fluoride help re-mineralize the tooth and create new layers of dentin.

In an article published on page 15 in the March/April 2013 issue of the Journal of the American Orthodontic Society, the article states that "Calcium and Phosphate must be present in Saliva with a PH ph between 7.5 and 8.5 in order for re-mineralization to effectively take place." Read the full article at:
http://jaos.orthodontics.com/publication/?i=153052&p=15

Your teeth constantly have a flow of minerals going in and out through them, much like a flowing stream. When your saliva has the proper PH balance, your teeth are naturally stronger and resistant to cavities. This is completely opposite to the way our stomach PH operates. In order for the body to properly absorb nutrients, the body's stomach is naturally acidic. This is because the gastric acid in the stomach breaks down the food into particles small enough to allow the nutrients to be properly absorbed into the body.

Chapter 21

Natural Cavity Repair Simply Explained

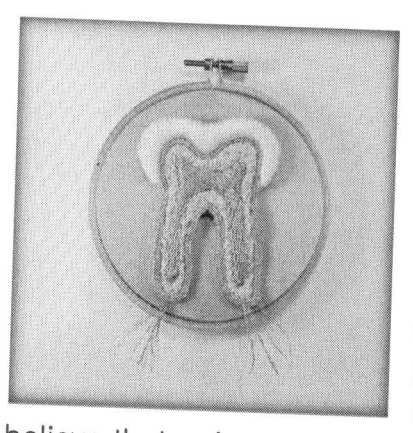

From my own personal experience, I personally have stopped seeing the dentist for the past 8 years. I sincerely believe that going to the dentist for fillings, root canals or other forms of invasive surgery is no longer a necessary part of my life. I personally for the last 8 years have chipped my teeth, gotten cavities, and had gum disease, at which time I easily "repaired" by simply eating the right foods, avoiding certain foods and/or taking intensive teeth re-mineralizing recipes.

Re-mineralization is a simple process by which you increase the amount of Dentin in your teeth. In some cases people have regenerated entirely new teeth, but I have yet to experience this myself.

Dentin is a layer that will form over the area of a tooth that is decayed or damaged. In some cases under the right conditions the tooth enamel also becomes re-mineralized.

Your tooth is made up of the following layers.

1: The Tooth Enamel.

2: Dentin the protective mineralized layer that's below the enamel.

3: The gum pulp. This area contains blood vessels, nerves and circulation.

4: The roots. These are coated with cementum, a tissue that is highly mineralized.

Dentin is the first layer that forms when a

tooth becomes damaged. The new dentin is deposited by special cells known as odontoblasts. Dr. Edward Mellanby states in the Journal of Nutrition and Disease that when the enamel and dentin of a tooth are injured by attrition or cavities, the teeth don't remain passive and just sit there, but instead behave just like antibodies responding to an infection or cut. They respond by producing odontoblasts in the dental pulp and begin forming multiple layers of dentine.

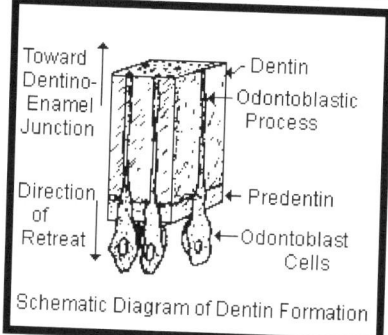

In 1922 Dr. Mellanby demonstrated that using varying diets of enhanced nutrition caused dentine regeneration in the teeth of animals both in quality and quantity depending on dietary factors. You can read an excellent summary of all the dental research of his work in a publication titled: Nutrition and Disease. The Interaction of Clinical and Experimental Work. Author: Edward

Mellanby. The book can be read for free from numerous sources online. Or you can read it as a PDF by doing an Internet search with the following phrase:
The Interaction of Clinical and Experimental Work + Edward Mellanby + PDF

Dr. Mellanby also did another study showing when a diet high in calcium, vitamin D and phosphorus was given to dogs, new dentine layers formed abundantly and rapidly.

This would explain why the average person on a diet with inadequate nutrition has to see a dentist if their diet does not have the proper mineral requirements. Most people's diets consist of diets high in sugars, artificial fats and white flour, which constantly form sugars in the body, creating a breeding background for bad bacteria in the body. Fermentable carbohydrates can cause sugars to form in the mouth. Foods that cause these include: white flour foods, potato chips, pretzels, cereals, excessive fruits and crackers.

How Amino Acids Help Reverse Cavities

Being vegetarian for over 10 years now, I supplement my diet with energy enhancing foods such as cottage cheese and carnosine. This allows me all the protein my body needs without the "bad" protein found in meats. After using Carnosine for the past 2 years, I had noticed that I did not have to do as many toothache prevention methods. I was also able to eat lots of chocolate (*up to 8 four ounce bars a week during the winter months*) and not even need to brush my teeth for up to a week afterwards. I ended up only brushing to remove the bacteria on the tongue that causes bad breath. I have concluded that this extra cavity protection is due to the amino acids in the carnosine. I hope that there can be some good scientific studies in the future showing that people who take a carnosine supplement have fewer cavities. The carnosine I use is an extra strength synergized form of carnosine that I mix with Spirlina. I call it the Overnight

Rejuvenessence Formula. The formula is as follows:

Just under 1/2 Teaspoon of Carnosine

1/4th Teaspoon of Brewer's Yeast
Just under 1/2 of 1/2 of 1/4th Teaspoon of Spirulina

1/2 of 1/2 of 1/4th teaspoon of Stevia Herb (Not the Processed Stevia)

1/2 of 1/2 teaspoon of 1/4th Mulberry (can use the mulberry powder from capsulated mulberry)

Grind the stevia and mix with ingredients and place into capsules with a capsule machine.

Let's explore the wonders of carnosine a little further.

The Miracle of Carnosine

Before reservatol entered the scene, carnosine was the #1 anti-aging supplement. Because Carnosine is an amino acid, it may be helping to rebuild teeth. Carnosine works synergistically with supplements that support heart health. These include vitamin D and Vitamin D3. I personally have noticed after taking the Carnosine RejuvenEssence Synergistic formula, that I have stronger teeth and gums. Part of this could be attributed to including the Vitamin D3, which synergizes with the Carnosine.

In a scientific study led by Jennifer Kirkham at England's Leeds Dental Institute, they developed an amino acid toothpaste. When it is applied to a decayed tooth, the peptides in the amino acids form a gelatinous scaffold that attract and holds onto calcium. This than allows the tooth to rebuild itself from within. The researchers than tested the amino acid toothpaste on a group of adults and concluded that the amino acid toothpaste reversed the tooth damage and regenerated the tooth tissue. What is interesting is my Overnight Rejuvenessence formula I use brewer's yeast, which is high in amino acids and

Spirulina.

In a scientific study titled: "A new biomaterial of nanofibers with the microalga Spirulina as scaffolds to cultivate with stem cells for use in tissue engineering" published in 2013, spriulina was used as a scaffolding for stem cell engineering.

In a study done in Russia, that concluded with a fully published 52 references, it concluded that "*Carnosine is a perspective immodulating tool which has many applications in medicine.*"

King's College in London published a review of the scientifically published carnosine literature, concluding with a record breaking 252 published scientific references touting the marvels of carnosine.

So we have over 300 scientific references attributed to carnosine. This means it must be doing something good for the body. Let's take a look at some of the many uses of Carnosine:

Carnosine has been made into Nasal Sprays, which allow faster absorption into the body.

Carnosine has been made into patches, which are used by athletes to enhance their performance.

Carnosine has been scientifically proven to enhance cognition in the elderly.

Chapter 22

Reviews of the best Toothpastes that Strengthen Tooth Enamel and Re-mineralize Teeth

There are some remarkable dental pastes available on the market today showing good remineralization effects. Let's look at some of the best. Many of these can be purchased on Amazon.com or other reputable merchants.

NovaMin – This paste will elevate your saliva PH into the 7.5 to 8.5 beneficial range necessary for re-mineralization. This allows the calcium and phosphorous ions to enter and heal de-mineralized teeth. Research has shown that NovaMin hardens enamel two times better than 5,000 ppm fluoride toothpaste. It also enhances fluoride uptake by 50% and can be found in products with 5,000 ppm fluoride.

The Complete Guide to Natural Toothache Remedies and Re-mineralization

Amorphous calcium phosphate – ACP decreases dentin permeability by 78%, which reduces tooth sensitivity. ACP will restore enamel luster and enhance fluoride delivery. You can find ACP in Age Defying Toothpaste made by Arm and Hammer.

Casein Phosphopeptide – When you add Casein phosphopeptide to ACP, it forms stabilizing qualities. Two toothpastes that have this are MI Varnish and Recaldent. Other toothpastes include MI Paste (GC America) and Trident Extra Care Gum. MI Paste includes fluoride forming calcium phosphate fluoride, CCP–ACFP. The addition of fluoride to Recaldent has shown improved remineralizing properties over CCP–ACP alone.

Clinpro 5000 – Made by 3M, Clinpro 5000 toothpaste contains tricalcium phosphate and sodium fluoride. 3M claims that Clinpro 5000 forms a harder, deeper layer than fluoride alone.

CaviStat – (an arginine bicarbonate calcium carbonate complex).

A scientific study titled: "*Clinical evaluation of the ability of CaviStat in a mint confection to inhibit the development of dental caries in children*". The researchers concluded that that CaviStat mint confection technology is one of the most simple and economical methods for substantially reducing the most prevalent disease in these children, namely cavities. CaviStat works because when the amino acid arginine and calcium salt is added to fluoride toothpaste, it greatly prevents dental cavities. In another scientific study, children who used CaviStat toothpaste for two years had 17.7% fewer decayed teeth and missing teeth compared to those children who used a standard toothpaste. The research study was performed by Colgate-Palmolive and published in the November issue of Caries Research.

In another study performed by researchers at the University of New York, Cavistat was administered in the form of breath mints and tested in a one year clinical trial and also proved itself capable of preventing dental caries in the primary molars and first permanent molars of children between the ages o 10 1/2 and 11 years old when the study was performed on Venezuelan children. The study was published in the Journal of Clinical Dentistry 2008;19(1):1-8).

Recaldent – RECALDENT™ is derived from casein. Casein is a phosphorous substance obtained from cow's milk. RECALDENT™ strengthens teeth by delivering the proper amounts of calcium and phosphate to tooth enamel. This greatly assists in tooth re-mineralizaiton. RECALDENT is available in Trident White Sugarless gum, Trident for kids sugarless berry gum and some other products worldwide. Because some of these contain aspartame, it is probably not a good idea to use the mints or gum long term, due to it being a possible carcinogen.

MI Paste U.S. Brand. GC Tooth Mousse (European Brand) – This product is marketed by the Japanese multinational dental products manufacturer called GC Corporation. In the U.S. it is called MI Paste and in Europe GC Tooth Mousse.

The good thing about GC Mousse is it contains Recaldent but does not contain aspartame. There are also several flavors to choose from. In an Amazon.com review, one woman suffering from extreme enamel erosion from receiving chemotherapy, used GC tooth mousse and after a few days of using it was back to eating normally. This was after her dentist tried a lot of other products. The GC Tooth Mousse was the only product that worked.

Pearlcium – This is a natural calcium obtained from pearls. A number of reviews from people using Pearlcium state that their teeth have improved after using Pearlcium.

Calcium Assimilation Formula – This combination is also known as Kid-e-calc (Calc Tea) Calcium Formula ("Dr. Christopher" products). It is manufactured according to the instructions given by the famous American herbalist John Christopher. It is a herbal formula that includes calcium combined with horsetail, nettle, oat straw & lobelia. It comes in 100 capsule bottles. There are also a lot of positive online reviews about this herbal formula as well.

Silica is an essential nutrient that scientists have recognized as being essential for bone health as well as the formation of healthy tooth enamel, fingernails and hair. The herbs Oat Straw and Horsetail and the food Oats (*oatmeal*) all contain good levels of silica, helping to strengthen teeth and bones. Cucumber also contains very high levels of silica.

Xylitol and Xylitol Chewing Gum – Xylitol is continuing to become popular due to its powerful cavity prevention properties. Many of Xylitol's advantages include fighting tooth decay, plaque build-up, bad breath and a dry mouth.

TriSodium Phosphate – Although I have not tried or used this method, there is a formula floating around out there consisting of 2 teaspoons of TriSodium Phosphate (TSP), 6 tablespoons of Baking Soda and between 16oz and 24oz of distilled water. This is than mixed together and shaken. You than swish this solution between your teeth for 2 to 3 minutes and spit out. This is done 2 to 3 times a day. This formula does make sense because Trisodium Phosphate (*also known as sodium phosphate*) is a powerful cleaning agent that is also used as a food additive, stain remover and degreaser. The white granular crystals are highly soluble in water and create an alkaline solution.

How to Use Remineralization Gels

There are a number of re-mineralization gels being sold on Amazon.com. So far the reviews and ratings of these have been pretty good. Many people are using these gels for negating the side effects of tooth whitening products or for sensitive teeth and teeth that have post bleaching tooth sensitivity.

Remineralization Gels require a mouth guard. You squirt a small and equal amount of the re-mineralization gel inside a mouth guard and place it inside your mouth over your teeth. The mouth guards are filled with the gel, left on the teeth for 20 minutes, then removed. Some people use re-minerlization gels so much that the gels lose their effectiveness over time. So it is best to not overuse them. If you decide to use a re-mineralization gel, be sure to read the reviews, instructions and user ratings carefully, as gels can vary in quality from manufacturer to manufacturer.

You can pick up mouth guards at any good sporting goods store. Just visit the Hockey player's section to locate the mouth guards.

All Natural Toothpastes And Powders

Uncle Harry's Remineralization Powder

This well known tooth remineralization powder has the effect of increasing saliva in the mouth. It works because as more saliva is produced in your mouth it becomes more alkaline, helping flush out debris between the teeth. This neutralizes food acids produced by the bacteria from eating sugary foods. The powder not only helps create an alkaline PH in the mouth, but also supplies the teeth with good levels of calcium and phosphorus.

Fangocur Mineral Toothpaste

This toothpaste contains bentonite clay, which as mentioned earlier in this book is a miracle worker at drawing out toxins from the sides of the gums, and helping fight infections. It is also packed with healing minerals. Fangocur mineral toothpaste consists of the following ingredients mixed with the Bentonite Clay: Essential Oils of: Krameria triandra, Citrus sinensis, tea trea, Mentha x piperita, Melissa officinalis, Simmondsia chinensis, Thymus vulgaris, Salvia officinalis, Curcuma xanthorrhiza, and Mimusops elengi. This formula is said to help soothe and strengthen the gums and provide minerals and trace elements to the teeth, helping re-mineralize them.

Chapter 23

Nine 100% All Natural Sugar Substitutes

At no other time in history since sugar was first introduced to the United States in the early 16th century, have there been so many healthy and natural sugar substitutes. Sugar can be highly addictive, however after using natural sugar substitutes, cravings for processed sugar fade over time, especially if you eat nutrient dense foods. From my personal experience, I have found that after using natural sugar substitutes for about 2 months, the natural sugar substitutes taste better than the processed artificial sugar.

These sugar substitutes I am about to share with you in some cases cost less, taste better than sugar and some of them promote gram negative bacteria (*the good bacteria*) in your mouth. These include Inulin Powder, Xylitol, Stevia or Agave

Nectar. I've added these powdered or syrup substitutes to plain yogurt, and the one that dissolves the easiest is Agave, however it does not go as far as Steevia does. This is because one leaf of Steevia can sweeten up to 5 or more cups of coffee.

Many of these natural sweeteners have about the same food energy as table sugar, but the best part is they won't raise Blood Sugar Insulin Levels or feed the bacteria that form plaques and cause dental cavities. Xylitol actually fights tooth decay, gum disease and reduces the ability of bacteria that cling to the teeth.

Maltitol and Xylitol

Maltitol and Xylitol have been scientifically proven to remineralize teeth [22]. Maltitol has shown to be one of the most powerful foods for fly longevity experiments. Fruit Fly experiments showed 100 percent of the fruit flies surviving 18 days when fed Maltitol [4a]. The average life of a fruit fly is between 40 to 50 days.

Stevia

The Complete Guide to Natural Toothache Remedies and Re-mineralization

Stevia is approximately 200 to 300 times sweeter than sugar, so you only need a little bit. Stevia is a 100% natural herb, found at many natural food markets. From my experience, a 16oz bottle of powdered stevia lasted almost an entire year. Stevia is also a natural probiotic synergist, complementing the yogurt or keifer giving the probiotics even more power. Stevia also promotes gram negative bacteria in the mouth, promoting healthy teeth and gums.

Agave Nectar

Another natural sweetener that I add to yogurt is Agave Nectar, which helps create good bacteria in the stomach also. Agave Nectar comes from a cactus type plant, and is about 1/3rd as sweet as Steevia. It has the same effect on the body as high fructose corn syrup, which can be bad or good depending on your lifestyle.

Cinnamon

Cinnamon is a great natural sweeter, and it helps lower blood sugar and keep inulin levels healthy. Steady blood sugar levels are the one thing that every person who lives over 100 (*centurion*) has in common. Cinnamon can also be very helpful in fighting the early stages of a cold or flu.

Inulin powder

Inulin powder is used a lot in baking and helps feed the stomach good healthy bacteria. Natural foods that contain inulin and increase gram negative bacteria include dandelion leaves, Jerusalem artichokes, chicory, bananas, garlic, onions and leeks. You can buy Inulin Powder from any good reputable merchant.

Glycerol

As a sugar substitute, glycerol has approximately 27 calories per teaspoon. Glycerol contains 60 percent of the sweetness of sucrose. This is because glycerin molecules are smaller than the sucrose molecules.

Momordica Fruit (also called Luo Han Guo or Monk Fruit).

Momordica Fruit has almost no effect on blood sugar and is up to 300 times sweeter than white sugar. It also has 5 percent of the calories of sugar.

Honey

Honey makes an excellent sugar substitute. I add it to tea and yogurt all the time for its immune boosting properties and the ability to increase calcium absorption.

Handy Hint: Calcium absorbs more readily into the body when taken in small amounts over a period of time, rather than taking large amounts all at one time. This means you will get more calcium in your body when eating small portions of cheese a few hours apart from each other.

Erythritol

Another natural sweetener is Erythritol. Erythritol is a sugar based alcohol used as a food additive. It was first discovered in 1848 by British chemist John Stenhous.

Lo Han. (Also called luo han guo or lo han kuo)

This powder is 250 to 400 times sweeter than sugar. It also has medicinal properties that include healing throat infections, coughs, heat stroke, constipation and diabetes.

Isn't it great that you can have an all natural way to have food taste as sweet as sugar, and at the same time promote gram negative bacteria in the mouth? Many of these natural sweeteners, after you get used to them, start tasting better than sugar.

Chapter 24

A Simple Diet Plan for Dental Health

While improving the strength of your teeth, avoid for at least a few days the following:

Sugar
Soft drinks
Excessive protein and salt
Chard, beets tomatoes, beet greens, potatoes, eggplant and bell peppers, excessive oatmeal

Eat more of the following;
Spirulina
Cottage Cheese
Sardines
Amaranth grain
Raw Organic Parsley
Watercress and turnip greens
Garbanzo beans
Leafy green Veggies
Seaweed

Besides getting an adequate intake of Vitamin D3, and I mean the D3 gel capsules not the powder because the gel capsules absorb better into the body. A major benefit of D3 is it also synergizes with Carnosine.

We all get cravings for sugary and flour based foods every now and then, especially when we are stressed or our diet is not high in the proper nutrients. It is okay to eat acidic foods every now and then. It is from an overabundance of acidic foods that leads to illness and disease.

An Overall Summary of the Nutrients that Create Strong and Healthy Teeth

After reviewing the large number of successful tooth rebuilding and strengthening formulas, there are a number of nutritional consistencies that constantly stand out. These are the basic and essential nutrients for teeth to heal themselves. Here is a list of the major nutrients necessary for teeth to heal themselves.

Natural Protein Enzymes (from Spirulina)
Stem cell enhancement (from carnosine)
Water
Phosphate ions
Magnesium
Calcium
Oxygen
Natural DNA stimulator (from amino acids such as brewer's yeast)

In a 2012 scientific study done by the Regenerative Medicine Group at Kochi University in Japan titled: "Branched-chain amino acid-enriched nutrients stimulate antioxidant DNA repair in a rat model of liver injury induced by carbon tetrachloride" the study concluded that branched-chain amino acid (found in brewer's yeast) stimulate DNA repair.

If you were to do a thorough search for a food or extract that contained the above nutrients in proper proportions you would find that chelated colloidal liquid minerals from ancient seabeds contain the above.

How to use Grape Seed Extract

I am mentioning grapeseed extract here because I have found it of extreme benefit for the upper part of the body. Not only is it one of the best antioxidants, but it also keeps teeth and gums healthy.

In a research study titled: "The antibacterial activity of plant extracts containing polyphenols against Streptococcus mutans", [34] researchers discovered that Grape Seed Extract reduced bad bacteria in the mouth that accounts for tooth decay. In another research study on Grape Seed Extract titled: "In Vitro Remineralization Effects of Grape Seed Extract on Artificial Root Caries" [35], researchers concluded that Grape Seed Extract assisted in remineralization of cavities.

Grape Seed extract also has many positive additional benefits such as slowing macular degeneration, relief of sore eyes from computer screens or glare, and reduction of myopia.

Test tube research showed that grape seed polyphenols inhibited the growth of Streptococcus mutans, which is the bacteria that causes tooth decay and that it slowed the conversion of sucrose (table sugar) into glucan, which is important for good dental health. It is also used to improve wound healing, improve night vision and is used as a cancer preventative. Grape seed extract is also a powerful natural anti-inflammatory. Usual doses range from 50 to 100 mg daily.

Grape Seed Extract Interactions; Grape seed extract can interfere with some liver medications. It also interferes with the common prescription medications: Phenacetin and Warfarin so use caution if you are taking these medications.

Chapter 25

Herbal Mouth Ulcer and Canker Sore Remedies

I mention this section because when I was younger, I used to get mouth ulcers all the time, and there were no natural methods to get rid of them and soothe the pain. In the book titled: "Herbal Medicine Healing and Cancer" written by Donnie Yance, he suggests the following formula for mouth ulcers.

30 ml Aloe Leaf Concentrate
30 ml Glycerin
15 ml Licorice extract
15 ml Propolis extract
10 ml Collinsonia extract
10 ml Echinacea extract
5 ml Chamomile extract
5 ml Thuja extract
5-10 drops of Clove essential oil.

The recommended dose is between 40 and 60 drops added to 1 to 2 tablespoons of warm saltwater rinse and used every couple of hours. The above extracts should be alcohol based.

A Remedy for Canker Sores and Dry Mouth

A formula named: Tooth and Gums Tonic, which so far out of 58 customer reviews on Amazon.com has received almost a constant 5 star rating is made up of the following ingredients: Essential Oils of Lavendar, Eucalyptus, Peppermint, Thyme and Cinnamon and extracts of echinacea and gotu kola. This is than mixed thoroughly with deionized water and vegetable glycerine.

How To Make Your Own Canker And Mouth Ulcer Salve

Apply a salve of the Essential Oils of lemon balm or licorice to the affected area to help assist in healing.

Chapter 26

Jakob Lorber's Second Sun Remedy

In Jakob Lorber's book titled: The Healing Power of Sunlight, he also talks about making a special salt that is supercharged with direct sunlight. Below is a chapter taken from his book titled: THIRD METHOD OF ABSORBING THE RAYS OF THE SUN. Seek to obtain a salt from which all mineral components, especially arsenic, have been eliminated. The best would be an absolutely pure sulfuric salt or a pure sea salt which would have to be thoroughly calcined until it no longer emits any visible vapor. Then it should be carefully pulverized. This salt, just as in the two previous methods, would have to be exposed to the rays of the sun for 2 or 3 months and also in a type of vessel as earlier described, preferably of a dark violet color.

When the salt is exposed to the sun it is of

importance that, several times during the day, it is stirred up well with a glass stick, specially made for this purpose. This stirring up or mixing is necessary because the finely pulverized salt would be lying approximately 4 mm high in the vessel in which it is exposed to the sun. So that all the salt particles at the bottom are exposed to the rays of the sun, the stirring must be done in such a way that not too many furrows or little heaps are formed. If this cannot be avoided, they must be leveled so that the sunrays can work evenly on the whole surface.

After such salt types have been sufficiently impregnated by the rays of the sun during the prescribed time, just as the sugar in. Heated up to a high temperature causing loss of moisture. The first and second method, they have to be protected from the effects of the atmospheric air in the driest place of the house, in dry boxes. When one wants to use it in case of some illness, special little spoons have to be made for this purpose, either of pure gold or pure silver, for taking out the needed quantity of salt. The tiny scoop must have a capacity no bigger than a lentil would fill, and this quantity is quite sufficient for adults. Children under 14 years shall be given only half of this quantity and children under 6 only a quarter. For this salt, especially the pure sulfur salt, has an extremely strong effect and acts particularly upon the bone structure, as well as on the teeth and hair, and is, therefore, to be used above all in cases of bone fractures.

If someone has broken a leg and the fracture is properly set and put in splints, it will be healed completely a few days after the salt has been taken. If it is a complicated fracture and the flesh and muscles of the leg are injured, such injury can also be treated externally, either with compresses of sunned water or with the well-known greenish arnica ointment, but 1 to 2 doses of the described salt must always be added to the water and to the ointment. However, for internal use, at the most 1-1/2 doses of this salt may be used even with the most robust person and it may be taken only once, for if it were taken more often, it would soon

bring death instead of healing.
Since it acts mainly on the bone structure, it would promote the ossification (bone growth) to such an extent that a person could soon become ossified in all his parts.

This shows the special effect of this salt. Properly used it heals, just as the earlier mentioned remedies, every physical disease, but great care must be taken. With the earlier shown methods, no particular damage can be done if the patient, considering his nature and the disease, is administered a somewhat larger dose or, if necessary, repeated in a few days. But with this salt there must never be a repeat, except after 10 years, and the dose must never exceed the prescribed measure.

The diet must be observed quite as carefully as with the earlier described methods. But the patient must abstain from sour drinks or foods for at least 14 days longer than with the other methods. This salt contains exceedingly intensive soul specifics, which are more or less also contained in every other acid, and it would initially attract the homogeneous soul specifics from all the other acids that enter the stomach and body, increasing them excessively, and the effect would be the same as if one already taken a double or triple dose in the beginning.

Furthermore, this salt has the effect, that if put on the tongue of a person near death, provided his organism is not yet too badly ruined, he can either recover completely or at least prolong his life span.

When properly used, it gives the whole body a proper current and gradually brings about a complete change in the body, so that after a year, nothing is left of the body the soul has been carrying around laboriously a year ago. Even teeth that people have lost are replaced, but the older teeth may become longer. Therefore, the doses must not be exceeded, as otherwise there may be trouble with a person's teeth.

Because Jakob was a professional, the salt remedy requires considerable caution.

The Complete Guide to Natural Toothache Remedies and Re-mineralization

There are also now commercial brands of these remedies available in both the plum ash toothpaste and the sunned salt. However use caution when using the sun salt remedy.

Jakob also states that the formulas work best on persons who are spiritually well-adjusted and whose bodies have not been subjected to unnatural foods, tobacco products, and the poisons of medicines. This would mean that people taking medications should use caution when taking the Jakob formulas due to possible interactions, much like the interactions that occur with herbs. The formulas work best with spiritually striving adults who consume pure, natural foods and also drinking several glasses of sun-cured water daily may enhance the benefical effects when taking the Jakob remedies.

Chapter 27

The Calcium to Phosphorous Ratios of Foods

Below are tables with the approximate ratios of Calcium to Phosphorous contents in various foods.

The Calcium to Phosphorus Ratio of Vegetables

14.5 -- Collards
7.5 -- Spinach, Mustard
4.5 -- Turnip Greens
4.3 -- Lambsquarters
3.2 -- Dill Weed
3.0 -- Beet Greens
2.8 -- Dandelion Greens
2.8 -- Chinese Cabbage (pak-choi)
2.7 -- Lettuce, LooseLeaf
2.4 -- Mustard Greens
2.4 -- Parsley
2.4 -- Kale
2.1 -- Chicory Greens
2.0 -- Spinach
2.0 -- Watercress

The Complete Guide to Natural Toothache Remedies and Re-mineralization

2.0 -- Cabbage
1.9 -- Endive (Escarole)
1.6 -- Celery
1.5 -- Purslane
1.4 -- Cilantro
1.4 -- Lettuce, Butterhead (Boston, Bibb)
1.3 -- Okra
1.1 -- Swiss Chard
1.1 -- Turnip
1.1 -- Chard, Swiss
1.0 -- Squash (winter, all varieties)
1.0 -- Green Beans
0.8 -- Lettuce, Romaine
0.8 -- Sweet Potato
0.8 -- Rutabaga
0.7 -- Endive, Belgian (Witloof Chicory)
0.7 -- Broccoli
0.7 -- Cucumber (with skin)
0.6 -- Carrots
0.6 -- Squash (summer, all varieties)
0.6 -- Carrots, Baby
0.6 -- Brussels Sprouts
0.5 -- Cauliflower
0.5 -- Kohlrabi
0.5 -- Pumpkin
0.5 -- Alfalfa Sprouts
0.5 -- Parsnips
0.5 -- Peppers, Green
0.5 -- Peppers, Red
0.4 -- Sweet Potato Leaves

0.4 -- Beets
0.4 -- Asparagus
0.2 -- Tomato
.02 -- Corn, White

Chapter 28

The Calcium to Phosphorous Ratios of Fruits

4.8 -- Papaya
2.9 -- Orange
1.8 -- Lime
1.8 -- Raspberries
1.6 -- Lemon (no peel)
1.5 -- Blackberries
1.5 -- Grapefruit, White
1.2 -- Grapefruit, Pink and Red
1.2 -- Tangerine
1.0 -- Pineapple
1.0 -- Pear
1.0 -- Apple (with Skin)
0.9 -- Mango
0.9 -- Watermelon
0.8 -- Cherries, Sweet
0.8 -- Grapes
0.8 -- Cranberries
0.7 -- Casaba Melon
0.7 -- Apricots
0.7 -- Kiwi
0.7 -- Strawberries
0.6 -- Cantaloupe
0.6 -- Honeydew Melon
0.6 -- Blueberries

0.5 -- Persimmon, Japanese
0.5 -- Raisins, Seedless
0.4 -- Peach
0.4 -- Plum
0.3 -- Nectarine
0.3 -- Banana

Chapter 29

The Oxalic acid Levels of Foods

Oxalic acid, a naturally occurring compound in many plant foods, can interfere with absorption of certain nutrients and deplete some nutrients, such as calcium from your body. The Oxalic acid level per 100 grams in Vegetables

1.70 g -- Parsley
1.31 g -- Purslane
0.97 g -- Spinach
0.61 g -- Beet leaves
0.50 g -- Carrot
0.45 g -- Collards
0.36 g -- Beans, snap
0.36 g -- Brussels sprouts
0.33 g -- Lettuce
0.31 g -- Watercress
0.24 g -- Sweet potato
0.21 g -- Turnip
0.21 g -- Chicory
0.19 g -- Broccoli
0.19 g -- Celery
0.19 g -- Eggplant

0.15 g -- Cauliflower
0.13 g -- Asparagus
0.11 g -- Endive
0.10 g -- Cabbage
0.05 g -- Okra
0.05 g -- Tomato
0.05 g -- Pea
0.05 g -- Turnip greens
0.04 g -- Parsnip
0.04 g -- Pepper
0.03 g -- Rutabaga
0.02 g -- Squash
0.02 g -- Cucumbers
0.02 g -- Kale
0.01 g -- Coriander
0.01 g -- Corn, sweet

Chapter 30

The Calcium Levels of Vegetables

309 mg -- Lambs quarters
210 mg -- Spinach, Mustard
208 mg -- Dill Weed
190 mg -- Turnip Greens
187 mg -- Dandelion Greens
145 mg -- Collards
138 mg -- Parsley
135 mg -- Kale
120 mg -- Watercress
119 mg -- Beet Greens
105 mg -- Chinese Cabbage (pak-choi)
103 mg -- Mustard Greens
100 mg -- Chicory Greens
99 mg -- Spinach
81 mg -- Okra
68 mg -- Lettuce, LooseLeaf
67 mg -- Cilantro
65 mg -- Purslane
52 mg -- Endive
51 mg -- Swiss Chard
51 mg -- Chard, Swiss
48 mg -- Broccoli

47 mg -- Cabbage
47 mg -- Rutabaga
42 mg -- Brussels Sprouts
40 mg -- Celery
37 mg -- Sweet Potato Leaves
37 mg -- Green Beans
36 mg -- Lettuce, Romaine
36 mg -- Parsnips
32 mg -- Lettuce, Butterhead (Boston, Bibb)
32 mg -- Alfalfa Sprouts
31 mg -- Squash (winter, all varieties)
30 mg -- Turnip
27 mg -- Carrots
24 mg -- Kohlrabi
23 mg -- Carrots, Baby
22 mg -- Sweet Potato
22 mg -- Cauliflower
21 mg -- Asparagus
21 mg -- Pumpkin
20 mg -- Squash (summer, all varieties)
19 mg -- Endive, Belgian (Witloof Chicory)
16 mg -- Beets
14 mg -- Cucumber (with skin)
9 mg -- Peppers,Red
9 mg -- Peppers,Green
5 mg -- Tomato
2 mg -- Corn, White

Chapter 31

The Calcium Levels of Fruit

49 mg -- Raisins, Seedless
40 mg -- Orange
33 mg -- Lime
32 mg -- Blackberries
26 mg -- Kiwi
26 mg -- Lemon (no peel)
24 mg -- Papaya
22 mg -- Raspberries
15 mg -- Cherries, Sweet
14 mg -- Strawberries
14 mg -- Tangerine
14 mg -- Apricots
12 mg -- Grapefruit, White
11 mg -- Grapefruit, Pink and Red
11 mg -- Pear
11 mg -- Cantaloupe
11 mg -- Grapes
10 mg -- Mango
8 mg -- Watermelon
8 mg -- Persimmon, Japanese
7 mg -- Pineapple
7 mg -- Apple (with Skin)
7 mg -- Cranberries
6 mg -- Banana

6 mg -- Honeydew Melon
6 mg -- Blueberries
5 mg -- Casaba Melon
5 mg -- Nectarine
5 mg -- Peach
4 mg – Plum

Chapter 32

Levels of Vitamin C per 100 grams in Vegetables

190.0 mg -- Peppers,Red
133.0 mg -- Parsley
130.0 mg -- Spinach, Mustard
120.0 mg -- Kale
93.2 mg -- Broccoli
89.3 mg -- Peppers,Green
85.0 mg -- Brussels Sprouts
85.0 mg -- Dill Weed
80.0 mg -- Lambs quarters
70.0 mg -- Mustard Greens
62.0 mg -- Kohlrabi
60.0 mg -- Turnip Greens
46.4 mg -- Cauliflower
45.0 mg -- Chinese Cabbage (pak-choi)
43.0 mg -- Watercress
35.3 mg -- Collards
35.0 mg -- Dandelion Greens
32.2 mg -- Cabbage
30.0 mg -- Chard, Swiss
30.0 mg -- Beet Greens
30.0 mg -- Swiss Chard
28.1 mg -- Spinach

27.0 mg -- Cilantro
25.0 mg -- Rutabaga
24.0 mg -- Lettuce, Romaine
24.0 mg -- Chicory Greens
22.7 mg -- Sweet Potato
21.1 mg -- Okra
21.0 mg -- Turnip
21.0 mg -- Purslane
19.1 mg -- Tomato
18.0 mg -- Lettuce, LooseLeaf
17.0 mg -- Parsnips
16.3 mg -- Green Beans
14.8 mg -- Squash (summer, all varieties)
13.2 mg -- Asparagus
12.3 mg -- Squash (winter, all varieties)
11.0 mg -- Sweet Potato Leaves
9.3 mg -- Carrots
9.0 mg -- Pumpkin
8.4 mg -- Carrots, Baby
8.2 mg -- Alfalfa Sprouts
8.0 mg -- Lettuce, Butterhead (Boston, Bibb)
7.0 mg -- Celery
6.8 mg -- Corn, White
6.5 mg -- Endive
5.3 mg -- Cucumber (with skin)
4.9 mg -- Beets
2.8 mg -- Endive, Belgian (Witloof Chicory)

Chapter 33

Vitamin C Levels per 100 grams in Fruit

98.0 mg -- Kiwi
61.8 mg -- Papaya
56.7 mg -- Strawberries
53.2 mg -- Orange
53.0 mg -- Lemon (no peel)
42.2 mg -- Cantaloupe
38.1 mg -- Grapefruit, Pink and Red
33.3 mg -- Grapefruit, White
30.8 mg -- Tangerine
29.1 mg -- Lime
27.7 mg -- Mango
24.8 mg -- Honeydew Melon
21.0 mg -- Blackberries
16.0 mg -- Casaba Melon
15.4 mg -- Pineapple
13.5 mg -- Cranberries
13.0 mg -- Blueberries
10.8 mg -- Grapes
10.0 mg -- Apricots
9.6 mg -- Raspberries
9.6 mg -- Watermelon
9.5 mg -- Plum

9.1 mg -- Banana
7.5 mg -- Persimmon, Japanese
7.0 mg -- Cherries, Sweet
6.6 mg -- Peach
5.7 mg -- Apple (with Skin)
5.4 mg -- Nectarine
4.0 mg -- Pear
3.3 mg -- Raisins, Seedless

Chapter 34

How to Make Your Own Zeolite Deotx Formula

Zeolite is a powerful metal detoxer from the body. You can usually find it in bulk or capsule form in health food stores. You can take the zeolite by itself with warm water or you can add the extra herbs shown on the following pages for an extra powerful zeolite mix, allowing you to use less. I made a small bottle that has so far lasted me almost an entire year.

Gather the following:

200mg of Lobelia or 1/2 a capsule,

1 to 2 cups of Raw Parsley (or 1/2 of 1/4th Teaspoon of Dried Parsley or the Powder), or you can soak the parsley in warm/hot water until the nutrients are extracted from the Parsley,

1 Vitamin C tablet (which synergizes with the Vitamin C in the Parsley). Vitamin C is also an excellent Metal Chelator.

1/2 of 1/4th Teaspoon of Lobelia (optional)

1/2 of 1/2 Teaspoon of 1/4 Cayenne Pepper (or just a pinch of the Cayenne Pepper is too strong), which increases circulation in the body to help flush out toxins.

1/2 Teaspoon of Zeolite powder.

Next mix the above ingredients and store in an airtight bottle. Drink zeolite with plenty of warm water for best results. Too much Zeolite is naturally extracted from the body and will not chelate any more metals if you take more, so it will only be wasted

The Complete Guide to Natural Toothache Remedies and Re-mineralization

Thank you for reading this book on natural methods to relieve toothache and have excellent dental health without pharmaceuticals or artificial substances.

I hope that this book can be a guiding light to those who want to learn how to properly look after their teeth. The information in this book contains information that either your dentist will never share with you, or has not heard about due to the lack of the resources to locate this book or the information all in one place. That is the sole purpose of this book, to have the best tried and proven remedies all in one place as a quick, easy and simple reference. Be sure to share this book and the information in it with friends, family and coworkers, as the more people can be informed about non-invasive methods to keep teeth strong, healthy and relieve toothaches, the less

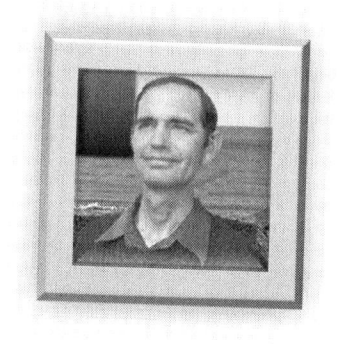

pain, money, time and suffering they will have throughout their life.

For every invasive cure there is always a non-invasive alternative. Many of these alternatives require a slight change in nutrition, and sometimes even for just a short period of time. Once the balance of proper nutrition has been re-achieved, invasive methods are no longer necessary.

Keep this book as a lifetime reference as you will never find such a complete resource on tooth health anywhere else.

Continued Life-Long Health to You!

Scott Rauvers

Author

The Complete Guide to Natural Toothache Remedies and Re-mineralization

Quoted Scientific References

(1)
The US Dental Amalgam Debate, 2010 Meeting of the FDA Dental Products Panel, Robert F. Cartland, Jr.

(2)
Parliamentary Assembly of the Council of Europe, Resolution 1816 (2011), available at
http://assembly.coe.int/Mainf.asp?link=/Documents/AdoptedText/ta11/ERES1816.htm

(2a)
Social, Health and Family Affairs Committee of the Parliamentary Assembly of the Council of Europe, Report: Health Hazards of Heavy Metals and Other Metals (12 May 2011), available at
http://assembly.coe.int/Main.asp?link=/Documents/WorkingDocs/Doc11/EDOC12613.htm

(3)
Health Canada
http://www.hc-sc.gc.ca/

(4)
Biol Trace Elem Res. 2013 Sep;154(3):326-32. doi: 10.1007/s12011-013-9743-3. Epub 2013 Jul 9.
Mercury transfer during pregnancy and breastfeeding: hair mercury concentrations as biomarker.
Marques RC1, Bernardi JV, Dórea JG, Leão RS, Malm O.
Universidade Federal do Rio de Janeiro, Campus Macaé, Rio de Janeiro, RJ, Brazil. rejanecmarques@globo.com

(4a)
The Newsletter of Longevity Books, West Towan House, Porthtowan, Truro, Cornwall TR4 8AX the Life Extension Foundation LONGEVITY REPORT 98
http://www.quantium.plus.com/lr/lr98.htm

(5)
Journal of Periodontology. March 2009, Vol. 80, No. 3, Pages 372-377, DOI 10.1902/jop.2009.080510. (doi:10.1902/jop.2009.080510). Relationship Between Intake of Green Tea and Periodontal Disease. Mitoshi Kushiyama,* Yoshihiro Shimazaki, Masatoshi Murakami and Yoshihisa Yamashit. Department of Preventive Dentistry, Kyushu University Faculty of Dental Science, Fukuoka, Japan. Correspondence: Dr. Yoshihiro Shimazaki, Department of Preventive Dentistry, Kyushu University Faculty of Dental Science, 3-1-1 Maidashi, Higashi-ku, Fukuoka 812-8582, Japan. Fax: 81-92-642-6354; e-mail: shima@dent.kyushu-u.ac.jp.

(6)
Antimicrob Agents Chemother. 2011 Mar; 55(3): 1229-1236. Published online 2010 Dec 13. doi: 10.1128/AAC.01016-10 PMCID: PMC3067078. The Tea Catechin Epigallocatechin Gallate Suppresses Cariogenic Virulence Factors of Streptococcus mutans▽
Xin Xu,1,2 Xue D. Zhou,2 and Christine D. Wu1. Department of Pediatric Dentistry, College of Dentistry, University of Illinois at Chicago, Chicago, Illinois,1 State Key Laboratory of Oral Diseases, Sichuan University, Chengdu, China. Corresponding author. Mailing address: Department of Pediatric Dentistry, University of Illinois at Chicago, College of Dentistry, MC850, 801 S. Paulina Street, Room 469J, Chicago, IL 60612-7212. Phone: (312) 355-1990. Fax: (312) 996-1981.

(7)
Prostaglandins Leukot Essent Fatty Acids. 2003 Mar;68(3):213-8. Pilot study of dietary fatty acid supplementation in the treatment of adult periodontitis. Rosenstein ED1, Kushner LJ, Kramer N, Kazandjian G. Arthritis and Rheumatic Disease Center, St. Barnabas Medical Center, 200 South Orange Avenue, Livingston, NJ 07039, USA. erosenstein@sbhcs.com

(8)
Antioxidant and Antiproliferative Activities of Common Fruits. Jie Sun ,† Yi-Fang Chu ,† Xianzhong Wu ,† and Rui Hai Liu *†‡ Department of Food Science and Institute of Comparative and Environmental Toxicology, Stocking Hall, Cornell University,

The Complete Guide to Natural Toothache Remedies and Re-mineralization

Ithaca, New York 14853-7201. J. Agric. Food Chem., 2002, 50 (25), pp 7449-7454. DOI: 10.1021/jf0207530. Publication Date (Web): November 9, 2002. Copyright © 2002 American Chemical Society

(9)

J Orthop Sci. 2000;5(6):546-51.Effect of combined administration of vitamin D3 and vitamin K2 on bone mineral density of the lumbar spine in postmenopausal women with osteoporosis. Iwamoto J1, Takeda T, Ichimura S. Department of Sports Clinic, Keio University School of Medicine, 35 Shinanomachi, Shinjuku-ku, Tokyo 160-8582, Japan.

(10)

October 1941. MASSIVE DOSES OF VITAMINS A AND D IN THE PREVENTION OF THE COMMON COLD. IRWIN G. SPIESMAN, M.D. Arch Otolaryngol. 1941;34(4):787-791. doi:10.1001/archotol.1941.00660040843010. Division of Nutritional Sciences, University of Illinois, Urbana 61801, USA.

(11)

Int J Cancer. 2007 Apr 1;120(7):1402-9. Inhibition of lung carcinogenesis by 1alpha,25-dihydroxyvitamin D3 and 9-cis retinoic acid in the A/J mouse model: evidence of retinoid mitigation of vitamin D toxicity. Mernitz H1, Smith DE, Wood RJ, Russell RM, Wang XD. Nutrition and Cancer Biology Laboratory, Jean Mayer USDA Human Nutrition Research Center on Aging, Tufts University, Boston, MA 02111, USA.

(12)

Med Hypotheses. 2007;68(5):1026-34. Epub 2006 Dec 4. Vitamin D toxicity redefined: vitamin K and the molecular mechanism. Masterjohn C1. Weston A. Price Foundation, 4200 Wisconsin Ave., NW, Washington, DC 20016, United States. ChrisMasterjohn@gmail.com

(13)

Study Title: Studies of anti-inflammatory effects of Rooibos tea in rats. Pediatr Int. 2009 Oct;51(5):700-4. doi: 10.1111/j.1442-200X.2009.02835.x. Epub 2009 Mar 27. Studies of anti-inflammatory effects of Rooibos tea in rats. Baba H1, Ohtsuka Y, Haruna H, Lee T, Nagata S, Maeda M, Yamashiro Y, Shimizu

T. Department of Pediatrics and Adolescent Medicine, Juntendo University School of Medicine, Tokyo, Japan.

(14)
Antioxidant and Antiproliferative Activities of Common Fruits. Jie Sun,[†] Yi-Fang Chu,[†] Xianzhong Wu,[†] and Rui Hai Liu *[†‡] Department of Food Science and Institute of Comparative and Environmental Toxicology, Stocking Hall, Cornell University, Ithaca, New York 14853-7201. J. Agric. Food Chem., 2002, 50 (25), pp 7449–7454. DOI: 10.1021/jf0207530. Publication Date (Web): November 9, 2002. Copyright © 2002 American Chemical Society

(15)
Cebrian D and others. Inositol hexaphosphate: a potential chelating agent for uranium. Radiation Protection Dosimetry 2007 127(1-4):477-9.

(16)
Crit Rev Food Sci Nutr. 1995 Nov;35(6):495-508. Phytic acid in health and disease. Zhou JR1, Erdman JW Jr.

(17)
Osborn, T.W.B. and J.N. Noriskin. The Relationship betwen diet and dental caries in South African Bantu. J. Dental Res. 16: 431 (1937)

(18)
A Comparison of Crude and Refined Sugar and Cereals in their Ability to Produce in Vitro Decalcification of Teeth. J DENT RES June 1937 16: 165-171.

(19)
Can Dent Assoc. 1996 Jul;62(7):578-84. Barodontalgia among flyers: a review of seven cases. Holowatyj RE1. Department of oral medicine and pathology, faculty of dentistry, University of Toronto.

(20)
J Am Diet Assoc. 2005 Jul;105(7):1071-9.
A diet rich in high-oleic-acid sunflower oil favorably alters low-density lipoprotein cholesterol, triglycerides, and factor VII coagulant activity.

The Complete Guide to Natural Toothache Remedies and Re-mineralization

Allman-Farinelli MA1, Gomes K, Favaloro EJ, Petocz P.
Author information
1 Department of Biochemistry, University of Sydney, Australia.

(21)
Climacteric. 2011 Oct;14(5):558-64. doi: 10.3109/13697137.2011.563882. Epub 2011 May 5.
Improvement in HDL cholesterol in postmenopausal women supplemented with pumpkin seed oil: pilot study.
Gossell-Williams M1, Hyde C, Hunter T, Simms-Stewart D, Fletcher H, McGrowder D, Walters CA.
Author information
1 Department of Basic Medical Sciences, University of the West Indies, Kingston, Jamaica.
http://www.ncbi.nlm.nih.gov/pubmed/21545273

(22)
J Electron Microsc (Tokyo). 2003;52(5):471-6. Remineralization effects of xylitol on demineralized enamel. Miake Y1, Saeki Y, Takahashi M, Yanagisawa T. Department of Ultrastructural Science, Oral Health Science Center, Tokyo Dental College, 1-2-2 Masago, Mihama-ku, Chiba 261-8502, Japan.
miake@tdc.ac.jp

(23)
Prev Nutr Food Sci. 2012 Jun; 17(2): 93-100. doi: 10.3746/pnf.2012.17.2.093. PMCID: PMC3866749. Dietary Intake Ratios of Calcium-to-Phosphorus and Sodium-to-Potassium Are Associated with Serum Lipid Levels in Healthy Korean Adults. So-Young Bu,1 Myung-Hwa Kang,2 Eun-Jin Kim,3 and Mi-Kyeong Choi3. Division of Food Science, Kyungil University, Gyeongbuk 712-701, Korea. Department of Food Science and Nutrition, Hoseo University, Chungnam 336-795, Korea. Division of Food Science, Kongju National University, Chungnam 340-702, Korea. Corresponding author. E-mail: rk.ca.ujgnok@76iohckm, Phone: +82-41-330-1462, Fax: +82-41-330-1469
http://www.ncbi.nlm.nih.gov/pmc/articles/PMC3866749/

(24)
Asian Pac J Trop Biomed. 2014 Jun; 4(6): 463-472. doi: 10.12980/APJTB.4.2014C1203. PMCID: PMC3994356.

Antimicrobial activity of some essential oils against oral multidrug-resistant Enterococcus faecalis in both planktonic and biofilm state
Fethi Benbelaïd,1 Abdelmounaïm Khadir,1 Mohamed Amine Abdoune,1 Mourad Bendahou,1,* Alain Muselli,2 and Jean Costa2
1Laboratory of Applied Microbiology in Food, Biomedical and Environment (LAMAABE), Aboubekr Belkaïd University, PO Box 119, 13000 Tlemcen, Algeria. Laboratory of Natural Products Chemistry, University of Corsica, UMR CNRS 6134, Campus Grimaldi, BP 52, 20250 Corte, France. Reviewed by Malinee Pongsavee, Ph.D., Associate Professor. Department of Medical Technology, Faculty of Allied Health Sciences, Thammasat University, Rangsit Campus Patumthani 12121, Thailand., Tel: Phone: 662-9869213 ext.7252, Fax: 662-5165379, E-mail: ht.ca.ut@peenilam. Comments: This study evaluated some EOs in treatment of intractable oral infections, principally caused by biofilm of multidrug-resistant E. faecalis. The results of this study is useful for E. faecalis infection treatment. The high yield and strong antimicrobial activity of three Algerian medicinal plants EOs used in eradication of MDR pathogens from oral ecosystem may contribut to the medical treatment for oral intractable infections caused by E. faecalis. Corresponding author: Dr. Mourad Bendahou, Department of Biology, Faculty of Sciences of Nature, Life, Earth and Universe, Aboubekr Belkaïd University, P.O. Box 119, 13000 Tlemcen, Algeria. Tel: Phone: +21343211572, Fax: +21343286308.

(25)
J Oral Sci. 1998 Sep;40(3):115-7. The inhibitory effect of funoran and eucalyptus extract-containing chewing gum on plaque formation. Sato S1, Yoshinuma N, Ito K, Tokumoto T, Takiguchi T, Suzuki Y, Murai S. Department of Periodontology, Nihon University School of Dentistry, Tokyo, Japan.

(26)
J Orthop Sci. 2000;5(6):546-51.Effect of combined administration of vitamin D3 and vitamin K2 on bone mineral density of the lumbar spine in postmenopausal women with osteoporosis. Iwamoto J1, Takeda T, Ichimura S. Department of Sports Clinic, Keio University School of Medicine, 35 Shinanomachi, Shinjuku-ku, Tokyo 160-8582, Japan.

The Complete Guide to Natural Toothache Remedies and Re-mineralization

(27)
October 1941. MASSIVE DOSES OF VITAMINS A AND D IN THE PREVENTION OF THE COMMON COLD. IRWIN G. SPIESMAN, M.D. Arch Otolaryngol. 1941;34(4):787-791. doi:10.1001/archotol.1941.00660040843010. Division of Nutritional Sciences, University of Illinois, Urbana 61801, USA.

(28)
Med Hypotheses. 2007;68(5):1026-34. Epub 2006 Dec 4. Vitamin D toxicity redefined: vitamin K and the molecular mechanism. Masterjohn C1. Weston A. Price Foundation, 4200 Wisconsin Ave., NW, Washington, DC 20016, United States. ChrisMasterjohn@gmail.com

(29)
Acta Biomed. 2011 Dec;82(3):197-9.Comparative study of cinnamon oil and clove oil on some oral microbiota. Gupta C1, Kumari A, Garg AP, Catanzaro R, Marotta F. Amity Institute for Herbal Research and Studies, Amity University, Noida, India.

(30)
British Dental Journal 199, 210 (2005). Published online: 27 August 2005 | doi:10.1038/sj.bdj.4812616. Title: Vitamin C intake and periodontal disease. A Borutta1 The Study can be accessed online at:
http://www.nature.com/bdj/journal/v199/n4/full/4812616a.html

(31)
Am J Clin Nutr. 1988 Sep;48(3):601-4.Comparative bioavailability to humans of ascorbic acid alone or in a citrus extract. Vinson JA1, Bose P. Department of Chemistry, University of Scranton, PA 18510.

(32)
Iran Endod J. 2012 Summer; 7(3): 127-133.Published online 2012 Aug 1. PMCID: PMC3467135. Propolis: A New Alternative for Root Canal Disinfection. Maryam Zare Jahromi,1,* Hasan Toubayani,2 and Majid Rezaei3. Department of Dentistry, Khorasgan Branch, Islamic Azad University, Isfahan, Iran. Dentist, Isfahan, Iran. Department of Oral and Maxillofacial Surgery, Isfahan University of medical sciences, Isfahan, Iran. Maryam Zare Jahromi, Department of Endodontics, Faculty of

Dentistry, Islamic Azad University, Khorasgan Branch, East Jey Avenue, Arghavaniye St., Isfahan, Iran. Tel.: +98-3115354123, Fax: +98-3115354053, E-mail: ri.ca.fsiuhk@eraz.m

(33)
J Am Soc Nephrol. 2010 Feb; 21(2): 261-271. doi: 10.1681/ASN.2009080795. PMCID: PMC2834550. Dietary Fructose Inhibits Intestinal Calcium Absorption and Induces Vitamin D Insufficiency in CKD. Veronique Douard,* Abbas Asgerally,* Yves Sabbagh,† Shozo Sugiura,‡ Sue A. Shapses,§ Donatella Casirola,* and Ronaldo P. Ferraris. Department of Pharmacology and Physiology, New Jersey Medical School, Newark, New Jersey. Endocrine and Renal Sciences, Genzyme Corporation, Framingham, Massachusetts; ‡Department of Biological Resource Management, School of Environmental Sciences, University of Shiga Prefecture, Shiga-ken, Japan; and New Jersey Obesity Group, Department of Nutritional Science, Rutgers University, New Brunswick, New Jersey. Dr. Ronaldo P. Ferraris, Department of Pharmacology and Physiology, UMDNJ-New Jersey Medical School, Newark, NJ 07101-1709., Phone: 973-972-4519; Fax: 973-972-7950; E-mail: ude.jndmu@sirarref

(34)
Caries Res. 2007;41(5):342-9. The antibacterial activity of plant extracts containing polyphenols against Streptococcus mutans.Smullen J1, Koutsou GA, Foster HA, Zumbé A, Storey DM. Biomedical Sciences Research Institute, University of Salford, Manchester, UK.

(35)
J Dent. Author manuscript; available in PMC 2009 Nov 1.Published in final edited form as: J Dent. 2008 Nov; 36(11): 900-906.
Published online 2008 Sep 25. doi: 10.1016/j.jdent.2008.07.011. PMCID: PMC2583354. NIHMSID: NIHMS77534. In Vitro Remineralization Effects of Grape Seed Extract on Artificial Root Caries. Qian Xie, DDS, PhD, Post-Doctoral Research Assistant,a Ana Karina Bedran-Russo, DDS, MS, PhD, Assistant Professor,b,* and Christine D. Wu, M.S. PhD, Professora,**
The Department of Pediatric Dentistry, College of Dentistry,

The Complete Guide to Natural Toothache Remedies and Re-mineralization

University of Illinois at Chicago, IL, 60612, USA
b Department of Restorative Dentistry, College of Dentistry, University of Illinois at Chicago, IL, 60612, USA
* Corresponding author: Ana Karina Bedran-Russo, Department of Restorative Dentistry, College of Dentistry, University of Illinois at Chicago, 801 South Paulina Street, room 551, Chicago, IL 60612, Phone: 312-413-9581, Fax: 312-996-3535, E-mail: ude.ciu@nardeb. **This author has formerly published under "Christine D. Wu-yuan"

(36)
Microbiol Rev. 1986 Dec; 50(4): 353-380. PMCID: PMC373078. Role of Streptococcus mutans in human dental decay. W J Loesche

(37)
PLoS One. 2014; 9(1): e87061. Published online 2014 Jan 21. doi: 10.1371/journal.pone.0087061. PMCID: PMC389776. Anti-Oxidative Effects of Rooibos Tea (Aspalathus linearis) on Immobilization-Induced Oxidative Stress in Rat Brain. In-Sun Hong,#1,2 Hwa-Yong Lee,#1,2 and Hyun-Pyo Kim3,* Xianglin Shi, Editor. Adult Stem Cell Research Center, Seoul National University, Seoul, Republic of Korea. Department of Veterinary Public Health, Laboratory of Stem Cell and Tumor Biology, Seoul National University, Seoul, Republic of Korea. Department of Biomedical Science, Jungwon University, Chungbuk, Korea. University of Kentucky, United States of America. #Contributed equally. E-mail: rk.ca.uwj@sssphk. Competing Interests: The authors have declared that no competing interests exist. Conceived and designed the experiments: HPK. Performed the experiments: ISH HYL HPK. Analyzed the data: ISH HYL HPK. Wrote the paper: ISH HYL HPK.

(38)
Can Dent Assoc. 1996 Jul;62(7):578-84. Barodontalgia among flyers: a review of seven cases. Holowatyj RE1. Department of oral medicine and pathology, faculty of dentistry, University of Toronto.

ADDITIONAL REFERENCES AND STUDIES

1. Magalhães AC, Wiegand A, Rios D, Buzalaf MA, Lussi A. Fluoride. in dental erosion. Monogr Oral Sci. 2011;22:158–70. doi: 10.1159/000325167. Epub 2011 Jun 23.

2. M. Vahid Golpayegani, A. Sohrabi, M. Biria, G. Ansari. Remineralization. Effect of Topical NovaMin Versus Sodium Fluoride (1.1%) on Caries-Like Lesions in Permanent Teeth. J Dent (Tehran) 2012. Winter; 9(1): 68–75.

3. Novel Anticaries and Remineralizing Agents: Prospects for the Future. JDR September 1, 2012 91: 813-815.

4. Nonfluoride caries-preventive agents Executive summary of evidence-based clinical recommendations. The Journal of the American Dental Association. September 1, 2011 vol. 142 no. 9 1065-1071.

There is an excellent study paper titled: "Sugar Alcohols, Caries Incidence, and Remineralization of Caries Lesions: A Literature Review" which has done an through job of showing the effects of many sugars and their effects on the teeth. This paper scientifically discusses that dental cavities can be reversed as long as they are detected and treated early on. It also discusses using Xylitol and how it can be used in cavity repair and tooth remineralization. It also discuses using the substance erythritol for lowering the incidence of cavities, as well as much more information. Highly recommended reading. The paper is listed below.

Sugar Alcohols, Caries Incidence, and Remineralization of Caries Lesions: A Literature Review. Int J Dent. 2010; 2010: 981072.Published online 2010 Jan 5. doi: 10.1155/2010/981072. PMCID: PMC2836749. S. Kauko K. Mäkinen*
Institute of Dentistry, University of Turku, Lemminkäisenkatu 2,

The Complete Guide to Natural Toothache Remedies and Re-mineralization

20520 Turku, Finland *Kauko K. Mäkinen:
Email: if.iknupuakisuu@nenikam.okuak. Academic Editor: Figen Seymen

Parliamentary Assembly of the Council of Europe, Resolution 1816 (2011), available at
http://assembly.coe.int/Mainf.asp?link=/Documents/AdoptedText/ta11/ERES1816.htm

Social, Health and Family Affairs Committee of the Parliamentary Assembly of the Council of Europe, Report: Health Hazards of Heavy Metals and Other Metals (12 May 2011), available at
http://assembly.coe.int/Main.asp?link=/Documents/WorkingDocs/Doc11/EDOC12613.htm

National Health & Medical Research Council, Dental Amalgam – Filling You In (2002),
http://www.nhmrc.gov.au/_files_nhmrc/file/publications/synopses/d18.pdf

The State of Queensland (Australia), Consent Information – Patient Copy, Dental Fillings,
http://www.health.qld.gov.au/consent/documents/dental_04.pdf

Health Canada, The Safety of Dental Amalgam, http://www.hc-sc.gc.ca/dhp-mps/md-im/applic-demande/pubs/dent_amalgam-eng.php Marcelo Tomás de Oliveira et. al., Effects from Exposure to Dental Amalgam on Systemic Mercury Levels in Patients and Dental School Students, Photomedicine and Laser Surgery (October 2010, Vol. 28, No. S2: S-111-S-114),
http://www.liebertonline.com/doi/abs/10.1089/pho.2009.2656

See Mercury Policy Project, Neurotoxic Effects of Mercury in Dental Nurses (7 September 2006), http://mpp.cclearn.org/wp-content/uploads/2008/08/fdadentalmppnorwayfinal0907061.pdf
Terry L. Meyers, When less is more -- Technology increases minimally invasive procedures, Dental Economics, http://www.dentaleconomics.com/index/display/article-display/6295266301/articles/dental-economics/volume-100/issue-5/columns/when-less_is_more.html (explaining that "with the resins and composites developed over the past 30 years, we don't have to remove nearly as much tooth structure as we did when using amalgam. Before these new materials with their bonding capacity came along, in some cases dentists

had to take out the whole back side of the tooth to get enough amalgam in there to work.").

Davis MW, Nesbitt WE. The wedge effect: structural design weakness of Class II amalgam. AACD J 1997;13(3):62-8, http://www.smilesofsantafe.com/pdfs/WedgeEffect.pdf.

World Health Organization, ART-Atraumatic Restorative Treatment, http://toxicteeth.org/CAPP-ART.pdf.

Christopher D. Lynch, Kevin B. Frazier, Robert J. McConnell, Igor R. Blum and Nairn H.F. Wilson, Minimally invasive management of dental caries: Contemporary teaching of posterior resin-based composite placement in U.S. and Canadian dental schools, J Am Denta Assoc 2011; 142; 612-620, http://jada.ada.org/content/142/6/612.abstract

See Bio Intelligence Service/European Commission, Review of the Community Strategy Concerning Mercury (p.229), 4 October 2010, http://ec.europa.eu/environment/chemicals/mercury/pdf/review_mercury_strategy2010.pdf

Zogby poll, http://www.toxicteeth.org/Zogby%20Poll--Results%202006.pdf .

N.J.M. Opdam, E.M. Bronkhorst, B.A.C. Loomans, and M.-C.D.N.J.M. Huysmana, 12-Year Survival of Composite vs. Amalgam Restorations, Journal of Dental Research (October 2010), Vol. 89, 10: pp. 1063-1067.

World Health Organization, ART-Atraumatic Restorative Treatment, http://toxicteeth.org/CAPP-ART.pdf.

WHO, Atraumatic Restorative Treatment (ART) for Tooth Decay: A Global Initiative 1998-2000 (1998), http://whqlibdoc.who.int/hq/1998/WHO_NCD_ORH_ART_98.1.pdf.

Pan American Health Organization, Oral Health of Low Income Children: Procedures for Atraumatic Restorative Treatment (PRAT) (2006), http://new.paho.org/hq/dmdocuments/2009/OH_top_PT_low06.pdf ("The costs of employing the PRAT [procedures for atraumatic restorative treatment] approach for dental caries treatment, including retreatment, are roughly half the cost of amalgam without retreatment.").

Pan American Health Organization, Oral Health of Low Income Children: Procedures for Atraumatic Restorative Treatment (PRAT) (2006), http://new.paho.org/hq/dmdocuments/2009/OH_top_PT_low06.pdf (The Pan American Health Organization concluded that its

The Complete Guide to Natural Toothache Remedies and Re-mineralization

"study demonstrated a higher cost-effectiveness of auxiliary personnel in some countries than traditionally trained dentists.") Jo E. Frencken, Evolution of the ART approach: highlights and achievements, J Appl Oral Sci. 17 (sp issue): 78-83 (2009), http://www.globaloralhealth-nijmegen.nl/ProceedingsTandheelkundeBiWe.pdf (finding that "a high level of acceptance amongst those treated with ART and an unwillingness to be treated again amongst those in the traditional rotary hand piece group [using amalgam].")
Van Amerongen WE, Rahimtoola S., Is ART really atraumatic?, Community Dent Oral Epidemiol. 1999 Dec; 27(6):431-5, http://www.ncbi.nlm.nih.gov/pubmed/10600077 (concluding that "preparations with hand instruments were smaller than those produced with rotary instruments.")
Frencken JE, Taifour D and van't Hof MA. Survival of ART and amalgam restorations in permanent teeth after 6.3 years. J Dent Res, 85:622-626 (2006), http://jdr.sagepub.com/content/85/7/622.full.pdf+html
Steffen Mickenautsch, Veerasamy Yengopal and Avijit Banerjee, Atraumatic restorative treatment versus amalgam restoration longevity: a systematic review, Clinical Oral Investigations, Volume 14, Number 3, 233-240 (2009), http://www.springerlink.com/content/ng3g624824682h53/
Daniel Zimmerman, Interview, Dental Tribune, http://www.dental-tribune.com/articles/content/id/3978/scope/news/region/asia_pacific. Proposition 65 warning, http://www.toxicteeth.org/CAPatientNotice2.doc

Index

Abscesses (Dental) 40,121,30

Ayurvedic 34, 35, 161,

Bentonite Clay 124, 131, 132, 184

Breath Freshener (how to make) 119

Calcium 20, 72, 77, 79, 98, 99, 106, 110, 113, 126, 140, 141, 147, 165, 170, 173, 176 Through 180, 184,189, 193, 204, 207, 209, 211, 213,

Carnosine 19, 61, 108, 111, 116, 171, 172 Through 175

Cell Salts 139, 141

Clove Vii, 21, 25, 30, 80, 106, 111, 114, 118, 130, 135, 196

Coconut Oil 21, 67, 68, 78,

Cod Liver Oil 17, 18, 21, 64, 65, 76, 77 Through 79, 82, 99, 99, 106, 107, 113, 138

Dentin V, 106, 165, 168 through 170, 177

Dentist Vii, IX, 14, 16, 167, 170,

Dew Point And Toothache 93

Dr. Weston A Price 16 Through 18, 64, 76, 81

Essential Oils 24, 26, 30, 50, 46 Through 48, 120, 130, 136, 149, 152, 184, 196, 197,

Eucalyptus Oil 47, 50, 65, 197

Fine Powder Herbs (Making) 45

French Green Clay 131

Ginger 25, 115, 126, 130, 154, 155,

Gums (Health) 18, 23 Through 27, 53, 57 Through 59,

Herbal Compresses 115

Homeopathic 28 Through 33

Horsetail 62, 63, 106, 151, 152 , 180, 181,

Hydrogen Peroxide 118

Immune System (Boosting) 71, 106, 122, 124, 135, 137,

Jakob Lorber 31

Jared's Tooth Powder 30

Jerthro Kloss 27,

Maltitol Vii

Materia Medica 44

Mercury Iii, Iv, 50, 53,

Michael Moore 28

Mouth Rinse 119

Native American 41 Through 43

Natural Tea 51, 54,

Niacin 123 through 124

Oatstraw 62 Through 63

Oil Pulling 61, 92, 97, 100, 102 Through 103, 109, 129, 132, 154

Ormus 59, 116 Through 117,

Parsley 21, 65, 70, 75, 79, 80, 97, 98, 112, 113, 124, 133, 138, 191, 204

Poultice 27, 30, 41, 42, 57, 60, 109, 116, 126, 127, 129, 132, 152, 153, 154, 157, 158, 160

Qucertin 92, 93, 107 Through 108

Rooibos Tea 61, 66

Sardines 53, 54, 58, 110, 191,

Spirulina 22, 62, 98, 106, 113, 138, 146, 153, 172, 174, 191, 193

Sugar 17, 69 Through 75

Sunflower Oil (Use In Oil Pulling) 18, 58, 77, 97, 102 Through104, 109, 112, 132,

Swedish Bitters 130

Sweetgum 43

Tea Bag (Use As A Poultice) 61, 132, 154,

Toothache Vii, Ix, X, 13, 19, 23, 25,

Toothache Immediate Relief Methods 31, 106, 111

Toothache, Causes 83

Traditional Chinese Herbal Formulas 28, 35 Through 39, 130

Tree Bark 31, 32, 43, 60, 65, 115, 116, 136, 137, 160,

Vegetarians 18 Through 19, 171

Vitamin A 19, 63 Through 65, 76, 80, 98, 113, 138, 149,

Vitamin D 19 Through 21, 63, 78, 79, 82, 108, 113, 148, 170, 173, 192,

Vitamin K2 19 Through 22, 63, 76, 78 Through 80, 107

Watermelon 44, 154, 155

Weather And Toothache 90, 92, 93, 95, 97,

White Oak Bark 31, 136

Yogurt 62, 75, 79, 98, 99, 106, 110, 112,

The Complete Guide to Natural Toothache Remedies and Re-mineralization

113, 133, 138, 186, 187, 189,

The Complete Guide to Natural Toothache Remedies and Re-mineralization

Printed in Great Britain
by Amazon